METABOLIC EFFICIENCY TRAINING

TEACHING THE BODY TO BURN MORE FAT

Bob Seebohar

Printed in the United States of America.

ISBN: 978-0-9842759-0-8

Bob Seebohar
coachbob@fuel4mance.com
www.fuel4mance.com

Design and layout by Kathryn Skiba

CONTENTS

PREFACE

I sincerely thank you for your interest in this book and appreciate the fact that you want to learn more about your body and how it can respond to different training stimuli and nutritional interventions. If you are anything like me, you seek new ways of improving and pushing your body to its limits while questioning conventional wisdom and science along the way. This could mean extrapolating sound research into practice, making theories based on current research or a little of both. With that said, I did want to spend a brief amount of time explaining my motivation for taking this information out of my individual consultation work with athletes and teams and bringing it to the athletic world as a whole.

Although I have been "around the block" and have experienced many things in my sports nutrition career, I still consider myself a student of the trade. I always will be. I seek more and more knowledge to help me understand the science and application of improving health and performance. I believe this is due to the ever changing processes within our body and the continual evolution of scientists attempting to answer their questions which then people like myself must try to apply to different sports and athletes or what I call "the real world".

I thoroughly enjoy asking the question "why" and believe it is one reason that I am able to implement and have such great success with the nutrition programs that I use with athletes. This metabolic efficiency topic has been my top priority to gather more information about as there is so much great application that it can have on athletes and their health and performance.

Before you sink your teeth into this book, it is important to understand that the basic concept of metabolic efficiency has existed for quite some time. There is published research to explain it and even to refute it, from an exercise intervention standpoint. There are still unanswered questions that exist in research, specifically the impact of nutrition and the periodization of nutrition upon these metabolic processes. I have been in the trenches with athletes for many years, developing the most useful and beneficial testing protocols to determine how to best use science to improve metabolic performance. The research on metabolic efficiency and the impact of nutrition periodization does not exist because individuals have not heard of the benefits these topics pose together. Institutions will not provide funding for studies like these because they do not see the health and performance benefits and thus the financial support does not exist. At least not yet.

No matter the reason, I have been using my ability and knowledge as an exercise physiologist and sport dietitian to seek the information that is in question. Through intensive literature reviews and real-life testing of athletes, I feel that I am at a point where I can begin to educate others in hopes that this metabolic efficiency concept can be developed even more in the future to improve athletic performance and the understanding of the human body under exercise interventions with different dietary manipulations. My goal for this book is to provide accurate background information about metabolic efficiency but more importantly, explain the impact that training and nutrition changes can have on it. Some of these data will be from my personal testing of athletes. It is not published in scientific research. I realize there are still some questions that remain to be asked and answers that I do not have at the current time but my passion lies in finding these answers through my continued work with athletes and the collaboration with my colleagues.

I hope you enjoy the beginning of the metabolic efficiency journey and throughout your reading, I encourage you to continually formulate your own set of questions and become your own experiment. I will provide you the tools to accomplish this and wish you the very best with your metabolic efficiency journey. I have manipulated and tested my personal metabolic efficiency for quite some time and have been pleasantly surprised at the results. My hope is that you will also.

Foreword

Nearly fours years ago when I first started training and competing in triathlons all the nutrition information I needed came from multiple sources in the form of literature, discussions and tips provided by other endurance athletes. It did not take me long to realize that the sport was driven by carbohydrates and at that point I did not see the need to reinvent the wheel so I got on board with that principle.

The energy roller coaster was part of every training session and even more prevalent on race days. I finished my first Ironman distance under a lot of distress, mainly gastrointestinal, and what I perceived as chronic fatigue. My race results over the next few years were satisfactory to most people standards but something was missing in order to reach the level of performance required to compete with top age groupers and validate my efforts by qualifying for the Ironman World Championships in Kona, Hawaii.

I knew that my training needed a little honing but my nutrition would require a complete overhaul. I attended a seminar on "Metabolic Efficiency" by Bob Seebohar and spent the next five months applying the principles he described. This "diet shift" included reducing my total calorie intake during training and minimizing the use of whole grains as a source of energy in my daily diet. I did this by shifting more of my calories to include lean protein, healthy fat and more fruits and vegetables.

The process was somewhat challenging at first but after the initial three weeks I could see and feel the changes. My body was becoming leaner and my energy level was increasing during Ironman training regardless of intensity and duration. The recovery was also accelerated thus allowing me to perform intense quality training sessions on consecutive days without jeopardizing the rest of my training schedule or immune system. Prior to eating more metabolically efficient, the day following a hard training session was always a struggle and it was usually a low intensity workout.

I recently raced an Ironman distance and my calorie intake was roughly 860 calories for the entire event which took me 10 hours. I did not have any stomach issues and my energy output was enough to earn a slot for the coveted Ironman World Championships in Kona.

Just imagine a race day where your nutrition is so simple and the related anxieties of mixing different drinks, gels and foods are eliminated. Imagine the preceding days leading up to a race without that bloated feeling due to increase calorie intake. For the first time in my racing career, I experienced this and would not change it for the world.

This metabolic efficiency shift made the most significant impact on my training, recovery and daily energy levels and I truly believe that Coach Bob has reshaped the approach of sports nutrition for athletes. Thank you Coach Bob.

- Alan Beauregard

Chapter 1
Introduction

The concept of metabolic efficiency came to me years ago when I realized that there was something missing from the sports nutrition services that I provided to athletes. I knew how to use nutrition periodization and implement behavior change and physiology testing principles into an athlete's nutrition plan but I felt like there was a missing link that, when discovered, would bring another level to understanding an athlete's body and manipulating it to achieve not only optimal performance but enhanced health. I sought to answer this question by tapping into the exercise physiologist in me and in a very short amount of time, I came up with the answer. Little did I know it would not be a simple "yes" or "no" answer.

I seem to awe coaches, athletes and sports nutritionists when discussing the topic of metabolic efficiency but in reality, this concept has existed for quite some time. I am not trying to reinvent the wheel. I simply did a bit of private investigative work to determine if traditional exercise physiology testing and equipment could provide some of the answers I was looking for to improve health and performance from the nutrition aspect and lo and behold, I found it! I have taken a known physiological principle and have brought it back to life to help athletes understand their bodies better. Metabolic efficiency testing takes the guesswork out of knowing if you are eating the right combination of food throughout the day or eating enough during training and racing. In fact, from one simple sub-maximal metabolic exercise assessment, you can easily determine the following:

1. If your macronutrient (carbohydrate, protein and fat) balance in your daily eating plan is in correct proportion to support health and performance.

2. If you are doing too much intense exercise too soon in your training program.

3. The number of carbohydrates and calories you need during different training durations and intensities based on your individual physiology and fitness level.

Metabolic efficiency testing allows you to accurately determine your body's nutrient requirements without having to depend on ranges found in research, or spreadsheets or formulas found floating around the internet. While these may appear to be helpful, they can grossly under or overestimate your individual needs. These ranges are fine to use when presenting factual, scientific data to large groups but they do not provide a customized plan for an athlete based on his or her needs. It doesn't matter whether you are an athlete, coach, sport nutritionist, strength coach or other health professional, this information is so applicable that it will be one assessment that will prove its worth over and over.

The combination of eating the wrong distribution of carbohydrate, protein and fat at inappropriate times of the year combined with poor exercise training methods can have a negative impact on metabolic performance. Most athletes follow some type of structured physical training program leading up to competitions and each training cycle usually has very specific physical goals such as improving strength, endurance, speed, power, technique and economy. Additionally, duration, intensity, power and pace are used frequently to ensure that the goals and objectives of individual training sessions are met. Most athletes prefer this type of planning and structure in their training because they have a method of tracking progress quantitatively. However, what puzzles me as a coach and sport nutritionist is that athletes do not put in half as much effort planning their nutrition as they do constructing their training plan.

Why is this so important? For the simple reason that the best training plan is worthless if the nutrition plan fails. This can lead to bonking, improper nutrient balance before and after training and gastrointestinal distress such as diarrhea, bloating, cramping or vomiting. This typically happens because nutrition is only given special attention a few days before competition which can be a recipe for disaster. Remember that varying your nutrition plan throughout the year will provide you the most benefits from a health and performance standpoint. Leave nutrition planning to the week before your competition and you are playing with fire.

Proper nutritional strategies implemented at certain times during a training year will provide you the ability to attain whatever your specific physiological goals are associated with each of your training cycles during the year. As I mentioned previously, each training cycle has different energy demands and physiological goals. It is important to understand these on a broad scale because once you have a better understanding of what nutrients your body needs based on your training, it is easier for you to manipulate your metabolic efficiency.

Chapter 2
Metabolic Efficiency Training

Efficiency is a term that is frequently used in sport. Athletes want to become more efficient because it is easier to move the body through different movement patterns while using less oxygen. From a nutrition perspective, being efficient means being able to use the proper nutrients at the right times throughout exercise and competition. It is about maximizing the use of some nutrients while preserving others.

Metabolic efficiency training (MET) offers specific nutrition and physical training recommendations to manipulate cellular processes that will improve the body's ability to utilize nutrients. Simply stated, the main benefit of MET is that it allows the body to use carbohydrate and fat more efficiently. This will have a positive effect on training status and health. We normally do not worry as much about the contribution of protein during exercise since it is not as significant of an energy source, thus, the macronutrients carbohydrate and fat will be the main focal points when discussing metabolic efficiency. Protein will be discussed later in the daily dietary manipulations.

Some athletes neglect the benefit of devoting a good portion of their physical training to foundational aerobic work for fear of not having enough time to improve their overall speed and strength. Aerobic training is often thought as less beneficial because the immediate physical benefits cannot be seen as much compared to when higher intensity training is done. However, neglecting aerobic foundation training in the preparatory cycle will typically lead to a decrease in metabolic efficiency because it can develop metabolic inefficiencies on the cellular level, which will have a negative impact on performance during the competition season.

Aerobic training plays an important part in this process because it induces changes in the mitochondria that improve the body's efficiency in using macronutrients, specifically fats. Mitochondria, which produce ATP (adenosine triphosphate-the energy currency of the cell), increase in size and number as a result of aerobic training. Mitochondrial enzymatic activity also increases. More specifically, those enzymes associated with the Kreb's Cycle and respiratory chain (the shuttle system that transfers protons developed through glycolysis into the mitochondria for use in the respiratory chain and fatty acid metabolism). I know, it's a little on the science side but the important take-home message is that through cellular adaptations, aerobic training allows the body to use more available fat for energy to fuel exercise.

The oxidation of fat by the mitochondria is the main source of energy when exercise intensity is low, typically defined in scientific research as less than 65% of maximum intensity. Depending on gender and size, an average person has about 1,300-2,000 calories stored as carbohydrate (commonly referred to as glycogen stores) in the liver and muscles and as blood glucose. Glycogen stores can deplete rather quickly (after about 2-3 hours of continuous training at moderate intensity) and carbohydrate supplementation may not be able to provide adequate energy for longer duration training due to the inconvenience of carrying or eating carbohydrate while exercising.

Additionally, athletes are at higher risk for getting gastrointestinal (GI) distress while eating during exercise because of the blood shunting response.

As the intensity of exercise increases, the working muscles require more blood and there is less blood flow directed to the digestive tract. When an athlete eats or drinks something under these conditions, the body often rebels and GI distress rears its ugly head in some shape or form. Think about it and your past experiences with GI distress and you will know what I mean. Was there ever a time (when you were not ill) that you had GI distress when you did not introduce anything with calories to your digestive system? Of course not because you had a "clean gut" and more importantly, it did not have to compete with the muscles for adequate blood flow. By reducing the amount of calories you need and therefore consume during exercise, you will have a much happier GI system.

Because of high risk for GI distress under exercise conditions, and the fact that the body has an excess of 80,000 calories stored as fat, it only makes sense to teach the body to become more metabolically efficient in using fat as an energy source. Use more of your internal energy stores from fat to fuel your body during exercise and you will reduce your risk of GI distress. It really is as simple as it sounds. From the testing that I have done on athletes, I have noticed that these metabolic changes can typically happen in as few as two to three weeks with properly implemented eating and training programs. In an ideal world, these training and nutrition plan manipulations should be done early in an athlete's season during the preparatory training cycle.

Aerobic training is important because it induces positive cellular changes as described previously but just as important is the quality of food eaten throughout the year to support your training program. Gone are the days where following the same daily nutrition plan is the norm. Nutrition periodization should be implemented throughout the year based on your goals, training cycles and competition seasons. Altering the nutrition program to support physical training and improving metabolic efficiency will complement your physiological goals of improving cardiovascular endurance, strength, power, speed and flexibility. These specific nutrition periodization strategies will be discussed in Chapter 5.

In addition to obvious performance benefits, metabolic efficiency training also has positive benefits to overall health. If you are not healthy, you cannot perform thus improving health should be the first and foremost goal for any athlete. Over-consuming carbohydrates, especially less healthy choices such as refined and processed sources, can lead to negative changes in your blood lipid (fat) profile, poor insulin control and the potential for weight gain. A high carbohydrate diet is linked with increasing levels of triglycerides (the main storage form of fat in the body). A high level of triglycerides (greater than 150mg/dl) is one of the factors considered part of the metabolic syndrome. Additionally, high triglycerides can increase the risk of becoming insulin resistant.

Insulin resistance is a condition where the body still produces insulin but it is not used properly thus the body's cells do not respond well to insulin. This leads to the body needing more insulin and thus it produces more but the pancreas, which secretes insulin, cannot keep up with the demand and excess glucose builds up in the blood. This sets the stage for developing diabetes. There is also evidence in research that shows that reduced levels of fat oxidation are associated with a high rate of weight gain and the inability to oxidize fat is a factor in the process of becoming obese.

As you can see, following a chronically high carbohydrate diet throughout your training year can cause problems from a health perspective and this can have a significant impact on your performance. Let me reiterate that I do not support following a seriously low carbohydrate diet. Neither end of the continuum will benefit you. Rather, meeting in the middle of the macronutrient range is the ideal and should be your goal throughout most of your training year. My goal for you is to adopt my nutrition periodization concept and principles to support your training demands, metabolic goals and good health.

Since we are not getting any younger, I feel that it is also important to highlight some research that has looked at the biology of aging and the impact on total daily calories. Many scientific research studies have concluded that as we age, calorie needs decrease and eating less may increase longevity. It is a very interesting concept and one that should be embraced by the athletic community. While there is certainly a time and place for consuming enough food and beverage to replenish glycogen and fluid stores lost during intense exercise, feeding the body calories in excess of what is needed on a daily basis may be a recipe for disaster in the long-term. I know, probably not what you wanted to hear as you may be one of those athletes who justifies their eating because of their training but it is at least worth mentioning. You should not approach your nutrition program with the "train to eat" mentality. Rather, you should strive to adopt the mantra "eat to train" and more importantly, your nutrition plan should be a factor in your long-term health goals first and foremost with using nutrition to improve performance a close second.

Chapter 3
The Crossover Concept

To fully understand the metabolic efficiency concept, it is first important to understand some history and background information. The crossover concept describes the relationship between exercise intensity and the use of carbohydrate and fat. It dates back to the 1930s and has been widely accepted among exercise physiologists with research to support it. Some of the many scientifically based explanations of the crossover concept include the following:

"Recognition of energy flux, as determined by relative exercise intensity, is the major factor in determining the balance of substrate utilization during exercise."

"Represents an attempt to integrate the seemingly divergent effects of exercise intensity, nutritional status, gender, age and prior endurance training on the balance of carbohydrate and lipid metabolism during sustained exercise."

"An interaction between exercise intensity and endurance training status with the net effect of these two opposing influences determining the relative contributions of carbohydrate and fat to energy metabolism during exercise."

As you can see, there are many perceptions of the crossover concept among researchers and, like many things in the scientific world, there is also conflicting evidence for the use and validity of the concept.

For example, it is argued that trained versus untrained individuals rely less on carbohydrate during high intensity exercise as noted from respiratory gas exchange data where training has been seen to decrease carbohydrate oxidation and increase fat oxidation even during intense exercise. The rebuttal states that energy flux, as determined by exercise intensity, is the major factor in determining the balance of substrate utilization during exercise. Additionally, supporters of the crossover concept indicate that the pattern of substrate utilization does not differ in trained versus untrained individuals as long as exercise is at the same percentage of VO2max.

The take-home message is to not get bogged down about which researcher or group of researchers adheres to a certain definition or theory but rather how they interpret the data and most importantly, how they use the data received from the crossover concept and metabolic testing as a whole. At the end of the day, definitions and theories do not matter as much as the application to you and your training and nutrition program. This is the main reason behind this book. To provide you the knowledge of how to apply scientific concepts to improve your health and performance.

As mentioned previously, the crossover concept (shown in the graph on the next page) describes the relationship of fat and carbohydrate oxidation to the intensity of exercise. As exercise intensity increases, the body prefers to use carbohydrate for energy. Most athletes know this; however, what is less known is that the crossover point, typically reported as a percentage of VO2max or heart rate, is the intensity where fat and carbohydrate intersect with the energy from fat decreasing and the energy from carbohydrate increasing. The basic message of the crossover concept is that they body prefers to use carbohydrate at increasing intensities while the reliance on fat significantly decreases.

The goal of improving metabolic efficiency is to extend the crossover point ("push" it to the right) as much as possible by teaching the body to use more of its fat stores at higher intensities. This will allow more area under the curve where a greater percentage of fat is being utilized at higher intensities. This will benefit any athlete in any sport of any duration both in the short and long-term.

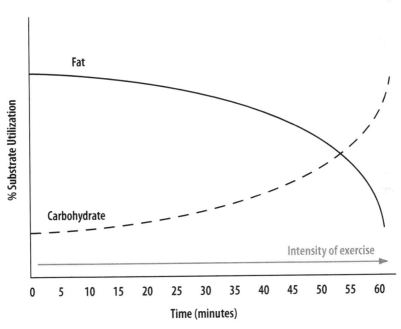

The Crossover Concept. The solid line indicates the percentage of fat usage and the dashed line indicates the percentage of carbohydrate usage during exercise. Note that exercise intensity progresses in magnitude as the graph progresses from the left to right indicating that carbohydrates are more preferentially used as the intensity of exercise increases.

Prior aerobic training results in cellular adaptations that can increase fat oxidation and decrease sympathetic nervous system activity. These adaptations can improve the ability of the body to use all of the energy substrates, but overall, the adaptations will favor more fat than carbohydrate oxidation. With higher intensities of exercise, certain biochemical adaptations contribute to the increased use of carbohydrate. Here is where I briefly jump into a little science so bear with me for a few sentences. These adaptations include contraction induced muscle glycogenolysis (the breakdown of stored glycogen to glucose so the body can maintain blood sugar and use glucose for fuel), increased recruitment of more skeletal muscle with a greater proportion of fast twitch fibers and increased sympathetic nervous system activity. Norepinephrine (similar to adrenaline which constricts the blood vessels and increases blood pressure and blood glucose levels) may stimulate both liver glucose production and lipolysis (the breakdown of fat stored in fat cells). Epinephrine (adrenaline) signals the heart to pump harder, opens the airways in the lungs and increases blood flow to the major muscles. This intensifies the contraction induced rate of muscle glycogenolysis which leads to a higher lactate formation. The acidic effect of lactate and hydrogen ion (H+) development inhibits free fatty acid transport by inhibiting a key enzyme, carnitine palmitoyl transferase, which reduces fat uptake into the mitochondria. Interesting stuff I know, but it is important to realize that there are some finite processes happening inside your body that contribute to you oxidizing more carbohydrate or fat as your intensity of exercise changes.

I refer to the crossover concept as metabolic efficiency and the crossover point as the metabolic efficiency point (MEP). I have found that it describes the concept better from the standpoint of broadening the understanding of which macronutrients the body is oxidizing throughout the continuum of exercise intensities. The crossover point, in my mind, limits the understanding of the application of the concept as a whole.

It is a common misperception that we only burn fat or carbohydrate during exercise. In fact, the opposite is true across most intensity levels. We are using a mix of both carbohydrate and fat to fuel exercise up to maximal intensities. The specific percentage contribution of each macronutrient will depend on individual characteristics, most notably exercise and nutrition adaptations. These can be manipulated with proper aerobic training due to the positive mitochondrial adaptations discussed previously but only if exercise intensity is maintained at lower levels at the right time of the training year. Training at higher intensities will improve lactate threshold, economy and possibly VO2max but will not induce macronutrient partitioning that improves fatty acid metabolism to the extent that aerobic training will. An athlete who is more aerobically conditioned can use more fat as energy at higher intensities and this can provide a glycogen sparing effect (preserving internal stores of carbohydrate).

Unfortunately, not every athlete has a textbook MEP. In fact, of the many athletes whom I have tested, very few achieve a MEP for one reason or another. The most common culprits include consuming too high of a carbohydrate diet or doing too much high intensity training at inappropriate times of the year.

Metabolic efficiency can be easily manipulated in a rather short amount of time which I will describe in Chapter 5. Some athletes and coaches have asked me if it is possible to predict an athlete's metabolic efficiency and MEP without formal metabolic testing. Although this metabolic efficiency "typing" is not impossible, I do not recommend athletes or coaches get in this habit because it will not provide the specific information relative to the ideal training or nutrition program that should be followed. For example, I can predict if an athlete will have a

MEP based on the amount of aerobic training in their exercise program, their physical training cycle and their daily nutrition habits but I cannot tell this athlete at what intensity their body makes the switch (if it does) to using more carbohydrate and less fat or what percentages of carbohydrate and fat that they oxidize. I cannot provide this quantitative feedback without conducting a metabolic exercise assessment. Similar to having a lactate threshold test, the information received from a metabolic exercise assessment is crucial for designing a training and nutrition program to improve metabolic efficiency since it is the specific intensities under the MEP that are important for enhancing the body's metabolic efficiency. Training at these lower intensities, reported as heart rate, power, speed or pace, will assist the athlete in improving metabolic efficiency. Although these lower intensities may be difficult to maintain at certain times, it is extremely important to adhere to them throughout the training year to induce the positive metabolic responses.

Here is an example to bring this to life. I asked an athlete whom I have worked with to have a metabolic efficiency assessment done so I could devise a more individual nutrition plan for her. I communicated with the performance center in her area regarding the protocol to use and she had the assessment done. I then asked for the data sheet and went to work. This athlete had a very clear MEP (at a low intensity) which was great but in order to improve upon this and make her more efficient at using fat at higher intensities, I communicated with her running coach the paces and heart rates in which she was most metabolically efficient at using fats versus carbohydrates. In her case, a pace of a 10:15 minute per mile or slower was her "sweet spot" for enabling her body to utilize more fat as fuel. This information was invaluable for her coach because he was now able to structure her run training to accommodate both her physical and metabolic goals. It provided him another level to his coaching that he had not had before.

What about lactate threshold you may be asking? Is there any relationship with metabolic efficiency? There is research that demonstrates the onset of lactate accumulation occurs at the same intensity as maximal fat oxidation. However, in the testing I have done, this is not the case in all athletes and many factors such as training status and daily nutrition can influence the results. At this time, I am not comfortable making the direct correlation between lactate threshold and the MEP for all athletes and do not recommend athletes jump to this conclusion as it may provide inaccurate training design information.

In addition to lower intensity, aerobic training, the MEP can be further manipulated through proper macronutrient partitioning and nutrition periodization. Eating a high carbohydrate diet leads to an increase in carbohydrate oxidation and the same is true with fat, although "fat loading" regimens have not been entirely supported in the scientific literature at this point as a performance enhancing tool. While the benefits of eating more carbohydrate may be justified during your competition season, this type of eating can work to your disadvantage at times because it will not allow your body to fully reap the benefits of increased fat oxidation.

Let me explain this in a bit more detail. Eating a high carbohydrate diet or eating a large amount at one time leads to an increase in carbohydrate oxidation. The body is efficient at regulating this in non-diseased states. However, this decreases the body's ability to oxidize fat due to the higher insulin response. As insulin increases, fat oxidation significantly decreases due to the hyperglycemic and hyperinsulinemic responses. Therefore, to properly teach the body to use fats more efficiently, carbohydrate intake should be maintained at moderate levels in the preparatory and transition training cycles and depending on the athlete, sport and number of competitions, possibly even during the competition season (I will expound on that a bit more later in the book and show you some case study data).

This is not a recommendation to follow a low carbohydrate diet. Please do not interpret it as that. As I will discuss in Chapter 5, the goal is to balance macronutrient intake so proper metabolic changes can be seen and since a large number of athletes eat an unbalanced daily diet, it is important to bring them back into balance and control blood sugar and insulin levels.

Lastly, it is important to note that other factors can impact the oxidation of macronutrients such as training status, blood metabolites such as lactate and free fatty acid concentrations, the proportion of type I muscle fibers, body composition and gender. Nutrition certainly has a large contribution but remember, we are talking about the human body which changes every second. Nutrition is only one piece in the puzzle.

Chapter 4
Measuring Metabolic Efficiency

Now that you have read and hopefully have begun to grasp the concept of metabolic efficiency, I am sure you are wondering how you can determine if you are metabolically efficient or if you have a MEP. While the testing protocol is quite simple, finding a location to have it done will take the most work because a special piece of equipment is needed to quantify your metabolic efficiency.

The piece of equipment necessary to assess metabolic efficiency is called a metabolic cart. This device can be relatively expensive, with the initial cost ranging from $5,000 to $25,000. Because of this somewhat large capital expense, it is more common to find metabolic carts in performance centers, hospitals and universities. Once you find a reputable location, the rest is easy! Well, relatively speaking. You just have to run or bike for a little while. Refer to the Metabolic Testing Centers across the United States in the appendix for a geographical listing of locations that provide this type of testing. It is not a comprehensive list but is one that I constructed based on a questionnaire that I sent out to various coaches and physiologists. It will at least give you a jump start in your quest.

One of the fantastic things about metabolic efficiency testing is that it can serve many purposes. It can determine your efficiency for using stored fat and carbohydrate, provide information on how to manipulate your training and nutrition plan to make improvements and it can help you determine a specific competition nutrition plan that is based on your physiology and current fitness level. I normally use the identification of the MEP during an athlete's preparatory season then as we move closer to competition season, I will use the metabolic assessment with a slightly different protocol to dial in their competition specific nutrition needs.

There are two types of metabolic assessments that are most popular: incremental and continuous. An incremental metabolic efficiency test provides information regarding the intensity (power, pace, speed or heart rate) at which the body uses fat and carbohydrate and when the "switch" takes place. It is the assessment that identifies if an athlete has a MEP or not with the protocol starting at a very low exercise intensity. It is important to begin here because identifying the MEP is the main goal and this will usually happen at lower intensities if the athlete is metabolically inefficient. You may not know if you achieve a true MEP if you are too overzealous and start at too high of intensity in the beginning of the assessment.

I cannot tell you the exact intensity level to begin since it does depend on the athlete's fitness level but if done on a treadmill, I begin most recreational athletes walking between 3.0-4.0 miles per hour (elite athletes will begin at a running speed) for the warm-up and note the trend of their metabolic markers. This will provide me an idea of their starting intensity. The athlete will breathe into a mouthpiece or face mask connected to a metabolic cart. The metabolic cart collects the breaths that are expired and will measure them for immediate data interpretation.

The ratio of the volume of carbon dioxide released to the volume of oxygen consumed is referred to as the respiratory exchange ratio (RER), also known sometimes as the respiratory quotient (RQ). It is important for the administrator of the assessment to keep a close eye on the RER during the warm-up and throughout the assessment as it is this piece of data that is extremely important to both end the test and properly interpret the test parameters and provide a useful prescription to the athlete.

Let me provide some information about this RER number. Different amounts of oxygen are required to metabolize carbohydrates and fat to carbon dioxide and water. The RER typically ranges from 0.70 to 1.0. The lower end (0.70) indicates fat is being used as the predominant fuel source and the higher end (1.0) indicates carbohydrate is being used as the predominant fuel source. As the intensity of exercise increases, so does the RER. The MEP is seen at 0.85, reflective of mixed nutrient usage.

HOW TO PERFORM AN ASSESSMENT: INCREMENTAL

It is important to instruct the athlete to fast (no calories or stimulants) for 2-4 hours before their assessment. After fitting the athlete with a mouthpiece and noseclip or mask (the latter is more comfortable for most athletes but may produce more error if a secure fit is not achieved), ensure the athlete is familiar with the exercise machine (typically a treadmill or bike) and understands the protocol that will be used. Instruct the athlete about the nature of the assessment, that being a sub-maximal exercise session. It is crucial that they understand that this will be a sub-maximal effort since the goal is to find the MEP, not go to maximal effort.

The athlete will then perform a 15-20 minute warm-up. Begin at a very low intensity relative to the athlete's fitness level. It is very important to keep the intensity low even though the athlete will want to go faster. You both know that they can go faster but that is not the goal.

The goal is to try to find the MEP if it exists and low intensity exercise is needed to do that. To perform a metabolic assessment on a treadmill, begin with the grade at 1-2% to best simulate outdoor conditions and increase speed between 0.2 and 0.5 miles per hour every five minutes. The athlete's fitness level will dictate how aggressive to increase the speed with beginners being on the low end and more experienced athletes being on the higher end. To perform the assessment on a bike, a power measuring device must be used and workload increases can range from 10-50 watts, depending on the athlete's level. Athletes such as elite cyclists can justify the higher power increases while beginner to intermediate level athletes will range between 10-25 watt increases each five minute stage. When it doubt, it is better to be more conservative on the speed or power output stage increase since the metabolic efficiency data at lower intensities is of utmost importance. Keep in mind that when using the treadmill, if an athlete goes from a walk to a run from one stage to the next, there will normally be a temporary increase in RER due to the physiological and biomechanical differences of progressing from a walk to a run. Keep an eye on the RER for a few minutes to note the trend. It will usually stabilize unless the speed progression was too aggressive.

The amount of time that the athlete should be exercising, not including the warm-up or cool-down, is roughly 35-60 minutes, or 7-12 five minute stages. This typically allows for enough data collection to provide accurate interpretation and doesn't allow the athlete to become too uncomfortable while wearing the headgear, mouthpiece and noseclips. However, if a continuous metabolic assessment is performed at a specific competition intensity (heart rate, power, pace or speed), an extended protocol can be used (more about this in the next section). It is important to remember that this is a sub-maximal effort only and taking the athlete to max is not necessary and is not recommended. In fact, the test can be stopped once the athlete reaches an RER of 0.92-0.94, assuming they had a MEP.

Interestingly, I have found that some athletes who do not have a MEP begin with higher RER's of around the 0.90-0.91 range. What normally happens is that the RER remains constant for a few stages but then begins to increase. In this situation, it is this increase in RER from their baseline that you would identify as the end of the assessment. Once the athlete is finished, include a 10-15 minute cool-down while continuing to breathe into the mask or mouthpiece to collect cool-down RER data.

HOW TO PERFORM AN ASSESSMENT: CONTINUOUS

After following the same initial athlete set-up protocol as discussed previously, instruct the athlete that the main purpose of this type of assessment is not to determine a MEP but rather to determine specific substrate utilization at a given intensity or a variety of intensities. The main reasoning behind this option is to simulate competition intensity measured as speed, power, pace or heart rate and measure specific substrate use during this time. The information gained from this continuous assessment will provide the athlete a more customized nutrition plan based on their competition goals. Most athletes whom I have tested will arrive knowing their intensity level at which they will compete, or will have a close approximation of it, thus the administrator doesn't have to do as much background work and calculation as must be done for the incremental method. It is always good to inform the athlete that this information will be needed before the assessment.

Have the athlete perform a 15-20 minute warm-up on the treadmill or bike while breathing into the mouthpiece or mask. Because finding the MEP is not the primary goal of this assessment, the athlete should perform their normal pre-competition warm-up which can sometimes include short efforts of higher intensity. Note the RER changes during this time for comparison when the assessment begins.

If the metabolic assessment will be performed on the treadmill, maintain the grade at 1-2% to best simulate outdoor conditions (this can be altered if the athlete knows the specific profile of the competition course). The speed should remain consistent throughout to simulate the athlete's competition unless the athlete specifies differing speeds based on their competition plan. While it will depend on the length of the athlete's competition, I normally recommend an exercise duration of at least 60 minutes for the run assessment.

To perform the assessment on a bike, a power measuring device is needed. Power output and speed should stay relatively consistent based on the athlete's predicted competition intensity. For example, if the athlete predicts she will maintain a power output of 200 watts during competition, 200 watts should be the intensity that is consistent throughout the assessment. Unless, as stated previously, differing power output tactical strategies will be employed during competition. Depending on the athlete's length of competition, I normally recommend an exercise duration of 60-90 minutes for the bike assessment.

Once the athlete is finished, include a 10-15 minute cooldown while continuing to breathe into the mask or mouthpiece to collect cool-down RER data.

This method of assessment is most beneficial in the

2-4 weeks leading up to competitions and throughout the competition season to continually fine-tune the nutrition plan.

ANALYZING AND INTERPRETING THE ASSESSMENT

Once the assessment is complete and the athlete has finished, the administrator can begin to analyze the data and "bring the numbers to life". While I am particular to a specific metabolic cart (ParvoMedics) to use for the assessment because of its excellent scientific validation and accuracy, a metabolic cart that measures both oxygen and carbon dioxide is adequate. The important factor is that the raw data be used in the interpretation. Do not allow a software program to do this automatically as it may not provide the information that is needed for proper data interpretation.

Many variables can be viewed and plotted together on graphs and in tables, as the data analysis is unlimited, but the following represents the more important variables needed to provide an athlete the applicable information regarding substrate use and metabolic efficiency from the assessment. Most importantly, it will show the athlete how to use the data in their training and competitions.

Time	RER/RQ
% CHO	% FAT
REE (kcal/min)	Heart rate
CHO (grams/day)	Fat (grams/day)

Important information needed to collect from the metabolic efficiency test to provide proper analysis and interpretation to athletes.

Legend: RER - Respiratory Exchange Ratio; **RQ** - Respiratory Quotient; **CHO** - Carbohydrate; **REE** - Resting Energy Expenditure

INCREMENTAL ASSESSMENT INTERPRETATION

As mentioned previously, the goal of this type of metabolic assessment is to determine if an athlete has a MEP and at what intensity it occurs. The information needed from the raw data sheet provided by the metabolic cart includes the percent carbohydrate and fat (%CHO, %FAT). Once you have this information, simply plot the these variables at each five-minute stage to show the MEP, if it exists. See the figure below for a visual representation (note: the example follows a "textbook" metabolic efficiency point and may not be experienced by all athletes).

If a MEP exists, it is easy to then determine the intensity (defined as speed, pace, power, heart rate or rating of perceived exertion) at which the athlete "switches" to using more carbohydrate and less fat for energy during the exercise session. Specific training zones can then be prescribed for optimal substrate utilization. In more simpler terms, the athlete will know what intensity to stay below to teach the body to oxidize more fat as energy. As the next step in the interpretation, an energy expenditure table can be developed which can help the athlete better understand their fuel utilization throughout the different increases in intensity.

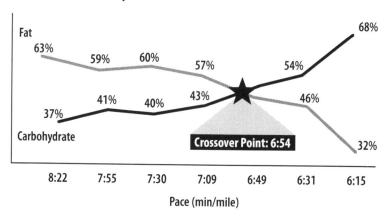

Plotting the percentage of fat versus carbohydrate to determine if a MEP exists. Each percentage indicates a 5-minute stage.

Below, you will see an example of an athlete's metabolic efficiency assessment with the information presented in an energy expenditure table format. Each column represents a 5-minute stage increase with the associated heart rate, calories expended per hour and minute, carbohydrate grams and calories expended per hour and fat grams and calories expended per hour. Providing these physiological indices assists the athlete in understanding their body's nutritional adaptations to exercise. Of course, more information can be provided but I would caution against including too much. Adding more data for the sake of simply showing it in a graph or table format may be overwhelming for the athlete and may not provide them the information they need to improve their metabolic efficiency.

ENERGY EXPENDITURE TABLE

Pace	Heart Rate	Kcal hour/min	CHO (gr/cal)	Fat (gr/cal)
14:16	103	355/6	18/72	32/288
13:20	128	495/8	28/114	42/378
12:30	137	510/9	33/132	43/387
11:46	143	528/9	30/120	46/414
11:07	145	536/9	31/124	46/414
10:31	153	578/10	38/152	48/432
10:00	160	580/10	41/164	46/414
9:32	165	621/10	50/200	47/423
9:05	171	650/11	63/252	44/396
8:42	173	695/12	90/360	38/342

By using this energy expenditure table, it is possible to provide an athlete the intensities and corresponding heart rates she is most efficient at utilizing fat. To do this she would view the last column titled "Fat (gr/cal)" as it clearly shows her most metabolically efficient intensities. Her optimal zones of fat expenditure range from a 9:32-11:46 minute per mile or a heart rate of 143-165 beats per minute. I would likely prescribe the slower paces and lower heart rate for her because carbohydrate expenditure is lower at these intensities. This will allow the most "bang for the buck" because it will act to "preserve" carbohydrate stores by not expending a great deal of them while maximizing the expenditure of fat.

No matter the applicable information that is shared, one thing is for certain: you can finally have a customized approach to your nutrition plan within the scope of your training session based on your physiology and fitness level. There are many alterations that can be made of the data. Again, find the most important one for you and begin to use it in your daily nutrition and training programs.

CONTINUOUS ASSESSMENT INTERPRETATION

A continuous metabolic efficiency assessment helps an athlete create their competition day nutrition plan with much more customization based on their individual fitness level at a specific point in their training program and accounts for the physiological and nutritional adaptations that were experienced during the previous months. It allows the athlete to dial in their training nutrition needs more accurately based on their own physiology rather than using the general calorie and carbohydrate ranges seen in many sports nutrition resources. Use the same information to plot the metabolic efficiency graph and create the energy expenditure table as you did in the incremental assessment interpretation.

The ratio of carbohydrate intake to expenditure certainly is not a one to one ratio. In fact, anecdotally, I have noticed that athletes who compete in longer duration competitions are lucky to be able to consume 35% of the calories that they burn through exercise. More realistically, I have noticed ranges of 15-25% as the normal "real life" calorie intake based on calorie expenditure. For example, if you burn 3,000 calories throughout a training session or competition, you would only be able to consume 450-750 total calories (using the 15-25% rule). What does all of this really mean? Quite simply it means that you burn more calories than you can eat. Think of it as an energy deficit situation. You simply cannot keep up with the calories that are being used by your body. If you try to eat more calories to keep up with the calories that they are being expended, it is a recipe for disaster, more specifically, GI distress. But remember, this shouldn't alarm you one bit. As you have been learning throughout this book, training your body to use more of its internal stores of fat to supply energy is the goal so you teach your body to need fewer calories during training or competition. You certainly do not have to practice feeding an enormous amount of calories to try to "keep up" with what you are burning. It is physiologically impossible and not needed. Plain and simple.

Because it will be quite an interesting example, let's take the energy expenditure table presented in the previous section and compare the carbohydrate (CHO) grams expended per hour at various intensities to the most updated, standard sports nutrition recommendations of consuming between 30-90 grams of carbohydrate per hour. What we notice is that this athlete has the potential to overeat quite a bit. For example, by looking at the 11:07 minute per mile pace, we notice that she is expending 31 grams of carbohydrate and 46 grams of fat at that effort. If this athlete consumed a modest recommendation of 40 grams of carbohydrate, she would be in an energy surplus condition, feeding the body more than it can potentially use during that specific intensity.

ENERGY EXPENDITURE TABLE

Pace	Heart Rate	Kcal hour/min	CHO/hour (gr/cal)	Fat/hour (gr/cal)
14:16	103	355/6	18/72	32/288
13:20	128	495/8	28/114	42/378
12:30	137	510/9	33/132	43/387
11:46	143	528/9	30/120	46/414
11:07	145	536/9	31/124	46/414
10:31	153	578/10	38/152	48/432
10:00	160	580/10	41/164	46/414
9:32	165	621/10	50/200	47/423
9:05	171	650/11	63/252	44/396
8:42	173	695/12	90/360	38/342

Additionally, based on what I mentioned earlier about the body's inability to eat as much as it is burning, she would be certain to be visited by the GI distress monster because she ate too much. This is a common occurrence in many athletes and I am telling you that you do not need to live with GI distress. Most of the time, it is simply a case of eating too many calories during exercise. Lastly, don't forget that in this example, consuming a higher number of carbohydrates would spike insulin levels and thus decrease the body's ability to use internal fat stores as energy.

Again, the point is that we can now individually assign a more appropriate calorie and carbohydrate intake based on knowing a little about an athlete's metabolic efficiency. Even if the athlete does not have a MEP, we still get extremely useful data similar to what is presented in the energy expenditure table. This allows us to manipulate calorie intake based on energy needs as their fitness level changes. This is truly an exciting time in the field of sport nutrition and exercise performance!

I understand that one of the first questions that may enter

your mind is if this is applicable for athletes competing in non-endurance sports or even endurance sports with competitions of shorter duration. It has obvious benefit and tremendous impact for any athlete competing in an event longer than 3 hours but would it be beneficial for events lasting less than 3 hours? The easy answer is "yes" but let me explain the reasoning since it is a bit different than for those competing in longer duration competitions.

During a shorter duration competition where intensity is usually higher, carbohydrates become an important energy source for the body. In general, most athletes have enough carbohydrate stores in their bodies to supply about 2-3 hours of moderately intense exercise (depending on what type of daily nutrition plan is followed). In shorter distance competitions and training, the primary two goals include staying hydrated and consuming enough electrolytes to promote a good hydration status and not rely too much on supplemental carbohydrates for energy. Yes, you read that correctly but before you jump to conclusions, let me explain further. By reducing the need for a high amount of carbohydrate per hour during higher intensity training and competition, as is often seen during shorter events, the risk of GI distress decreases significantly. Remember as I explained before, every opportunity in which your digestive tract must process calories at higher intensities, the greater risk of GI distress. What about athletes who engage in contact with other athletes such as seen in combat sports? These athletes often do not eat anything during competition for fear that they will get hit and vomit. A clean gut is very important in this situation. Overfeeding calories during higher intensity exercise is a recipe for disaster for most athletes.

Thus, by teaching the body to use its internal fat stores more efficiently in the early part of the training year and continuing to support this metabolic change throughout the competition season, more fat can be used as fuel at higher intensities and thereby reduce the need for high carbohydrate consumption. This does not mean supplemental carbohydrates are not needed. They are but when implemented properly, this metabolic efficiency plan will reduce your reliance on supplemental carbohydrates. It simply means that less is more because the body will rely more on its fat stores for energy and preserve internal carbohydrate stores a bit longer. That, in the short and long-term, is extremely beneficial for any athlete and I will discuss the steps to accomplish this in the next chapter.

As I conclude this chapter the take-home message is that you should work to improve your body's ability to use fat at lower and higher intensities. This will benefit you from an energy standpoint in addition to reducing your risk of GI distress. You do not need to overfeed your body carbohydrates during training or competition in an effort to train it to absorb more.

Chapter 5
Periodization Planning and Metabolic Efficiency

I am sure the first four chapters have gotten you very excited about the metabolic efficiency concept and if you are like most athletes whom I have worked with, you want to know how to finally put it together and reap the benefits. I thank you for your patience and for diligently reading the first four chapters to gain the ever important background knowledge on the topic. Now, let's get started with the implementation strategies.

Step one in improving metabolic efficiency is to periodize your carbohydrate intake as your training volume and intensity changes. Carbohydrates are a staple in any athlete's eating plan and for good reason. They provide the energy that is needed to fuel the body for training sessions and to fuel the brain for cognitive functioning. However, during certain times of the training year, maintaining a higher carbohydrate daily eating plan can work against your metabolic efficiency goals. When you eat too many carbohydrates, the other macronutrients, protein and fat, fall well below what is needed to support training and this can be problematic and become the catalyst for metabolic inefficiency. As you learned previously, eating carbohydrate leads to an increase in carbohydrate oxidation. I encourage you to use the concept of nutrition periodization and apply it to your metabolic efficiency goals throughout the year. Your nutrition needs will change based on your goals for your competition season, body composition and weight, the number and type of competitions that you have and the duration of your competitions. Thus it is important to factor in when it is most beneficial for you to oxidize more fat or carbohydrate for energy.

Step two in improving metabolic efficiency is to include aerobic exercise in your training program. The concept of physical periodization (separating your training into different cycles throughout the year) has existed for decades. The most popular periodization plan is a linear progression model that begins with improving aerobic endurance and strength, building speed and economy, peaking for competitions then settling down after the season for a well-deserved mental and physical break (the off-season).

This type of progression works very well for improving metabolic efficiency because during the preparatory training cycle, improving aerobic endurance is normally the primary goal. This is usually accomplished with lower intensity and possibly longer duration training. It is this type of aerobic training that will provide the most benefit to improving the cellular processes of improving fat oxidation. When intensity begins to increase too much without a strong aerobic foundation, the cellular responses favor carbohydrate oxidation thus the body minimizes its fat use.

With that introduction, it is time to provide specific recommendations of improving and maintaining metabolic efficiency based on the training cycles in which you will likely progress throughout the year.

PREPARATORY (ALSO CALLED BASE OR PRESEASON) CYCLE METABOLIC EFFICIENCY PLANNING

There isn't one particular time of the year where improving metabolic efficiency must be done or else it won't work. However, there are times of the year when it is easier to manipulate your metabolic efficiency without having to make compromises in your training. The majority of athletes will begin their training year by gradually introducing volume and intensity in a linear manner. This training cycle usually contains mostly aerobic sessions which makes this a key time of the year to teach the body to use more of its fat stores.

Remember as you read through this chapter that the two steps for improving metabolic efficiency are periodizing nutrient intake and training aerobically. The following are my recommendations for the preparatory training cycle.

NUTRITION STRATEGIES

By far the most important nutritional intervention you can make is to balance your daily macronutrient intake so it favors a mix of "healthy" carbohydrates, lean protein and beneficial fat. More specifically, focus on having a lean protein, healthy fat (omega-3 fat is most preferable) and fruit and/or vegetable at every feeding (I define a feeding as a meal or snack).

Minimize your whole grain intake as much as possible as you do not need as many carbohydrates since your training volume and intensity is not too high. In fact, challenge yourself and try not to eat any whole grains. I know it may be extremely difficult to do this as it may be engrained in your habits but it will benefit your metabolic efficiency in the long run. Don't worry about not getting enough carbohydrates. You will get all of the carbohydrates your brain, muscles and liver needs from fruits, vegetables, beans, nuts and dairy products.

Do not, I repeat, do not consume any sports nutrition products that contain calories (sports drinks, gels, bars, chews, etc.) throughout the day or before, during or after training. These products are formulated to supply nutrients when the body needs it most and this is not the time. Far too many athletes depend on these products when they first begin training again after their off-season and using them is simply a waste of calories and can lead to metabolic inefficiency. Just because you have increased your training from the off-season does not mean you should justify using these products for any training session that is less than 2-3 hours in duration. In fact, I wouldn't use them at all until the next training cycle. I know, this recommendation is completely different than what you may be used to or than your training partners follow but trust me, you do not need these just yet. Do not justify the use of these products as a reward for beginning a training program again. This is usually associated with unwanted weight gain, not to mention starting off on the wrong foot by not teaching the body to utilize its fat stores.

How are you supposed to fuel your workouts if you shouldn't use sports nutrition products? Simple. Depend on your daily eating plan and whole foods to satisfy your nutrient needs. The key to improving metabolic efficiency is having a small feeding that is well-balanced (not comprised of all high carbohydrate foods but one that includes lean protein and healthy fat) in the hour or two leading up to your training session to ensure that you are not "turning off" your fat burning processes. No bagels, pasta or oatmeal. Sorry. The goal is to achieve balance so add a good helping of chicken or salmon to a large spinach salad with veggies or spoon in some berries with some plain yogurt and extra virgin olive oil to make your feedings more metabolically efficient. I know this may seem a bit awkward as it does not support the normal thinking of consuming a high carbohydrate food before training but eating too many carbohydrates without protein or fat can spike your blood insulin thereby significantly reducing your body's ability to oxidize fat.

Consume only water and electrolytes (if needed) during a training session. Yes, you heard me correctly. This will, without a doubt, challenge your normal paradigm of thinking but remember that the goal is to improve your body's ability to oxidize fat. As you learned earlier, eating carbohydrates promotes their oxidation. To drive the point home once more, remember that the increase in insulin, in response to a high carbohydrate feeding (especially from simple sugars found in many sports nutrition products), will significantly decrease fat oxidation. Of course, the reason this is implemented in this training cycle is because volume of training should not be too high yet so you will be able to sustain training by focusing only on fluid intake and possibly electrolyte supplementation during training. You will need some form of carbohydrates as your volume and intensity increase but until that happens, there is simply no need for carbohydrate supplementation during training if you properly time your nutrient intake beforehand.

Here comes yet another surprise. It is not as important to eat for "recovery" after most training sessions during this cycle. If the majority of your training is predominantly aerobic with very little, if any, intensity and you do not have workouts that are glycogen depleting (as defined as longer than 3 hours or of high intensity), there is simply no need to eat to "recover" after training sessions. Focus on consuming water and some electrolytes to start the rehydration process and possibly a light feeding that is balanced with lean protein, healthy fat such as omega-3's and fruits or vegetables. There is no need for sports nutrition products after these types of workouts nor should you gorge yourself with a high amount of calories. A great tip is if you can try to plan your training sessions around meal times so you can easily use food in the before and after windows of training without overfeeding your body. In fact, I often recommend athletes make a little more of a metabolically efficient feeding before a training session and consume half of it before and half of it afterwards if they are hungry. However, that being said, it is important to mention that balancing your blood sugar and insulin levels will create adaptations in your body that you will not be used to. Once metabolically efficient, you will not crave a large amount of food in the post-workout window. This is a very good sign and one that you should eagerly anticipate.

I know you may be asking how much of each nutrient you should eat and I understand this concern because media has brainwashed you into thinking that counting calories is important. I am here to tell you that it is not, at least in the early stages of becoming more metabolically efficient through your daily nutrition habits.

I will not provide quantitative information concerning grams, calories or serving size recommendations in this book and this is on purpose. If you can focus most of your feedings on what I mentioned previously by including portions of lean protein, healthy fat and fruits or vegetables, you will improve your satiety (feeling of fullness). Because I truly believe in the "simple is sustainable" approach with athletes, I do not want you to get bogged down by measuring food or counting calories. I want you to spend your time focusing on what types of responses you receive from your body after eating certain foods. Clue in to your hunger and satiety responses and you will be more successful with this lifestyle intervention.

When you feed yourself, make sure to have sources of protein, fiber and fat and you will quickly notice how easy it is to maintain your fullness for at least three hours. A good rule of thumb is if you get hungry throughout the day and it has been less than three hours between feedings, your nutrient partitioning was a bit off. To improve this, simply add a few more bites of lean protein with fiber rich food (fruits and vegetables) with a dash of healthy fat and you will notice an immediate impact. Keep in mind that it usually takes a few days to get re-acquainted with your body signals and hunger cues again so be patient. You may under-eat and overeat in this timeframe but for good reason as you are learning the instinctual aspect of biological hunger once again. Learn your instincts, listen to them, then trust them.

To make it ever easier for you, I have created my Periodization Plates™. As you can see from the graphic on the next page, you can use your plate as a reference point for food partitioning. I know it sounds confusing but in reality, there is nothing more simple. By using my Periodization Plates™, you can easily navigate what type and the quantity of food to put on your plate based on your metabolic efficiency goals. I have separated the Periodization Plates™ into four easy phases depending on your training cycles. This again stresses the importance of approaching your nutrition intake based on your physical training goals throughout the year. Please do not get too obsessive about making your plate look exactly like one of my Periodization Plates™. That is not the point and that would defeat their purpose. Use them as your guide, especially in the beginning of your journey, to assist you in implementing the metabolic efficiency concept. They will be a tremendous help and as you progress, decide which plate may best suit your needs and how you may manipulate your plate to fit your individual goals and taste preferences.

Periodization Plates™

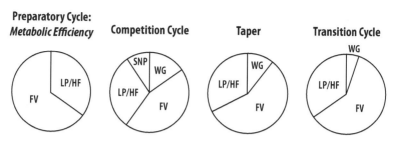

LP/HF: Lean Protein and Healthy Fats
FV: Fruits and Vegetables
WG: Whole Grains
SNP: Sports Nutrition Products

TRAINING STRATEGIES

If you are following a traditional training periodization plan that focuses on a gradual increase in volume and intensity please stay in your aerobic training zones for the majority of your training. That is the best piece of advice I can give as it relates to your training plan. If you have done a lactate threshold test, you know exactly what heart rates, power, pace or speed zones this correlates with and I encourage you to adhere to these lower intensity training zones. You can also use your breathing rate and conversation as a marker of staying aerobic. You should not be panting or unable to construct a short sentence while exercising. I understand that this may be a very difficult task to accomplish 100% of the time because you are most likely excited to get back into training and you have a great competition season planned. However, keep in mind your metabolic efficiency goals and take this small amount of time to improve your body's use of fats as it will provide you tremendous benefit when you start your higher intensity training and as you progress into your competition season.

You certainly do not have to partake in low intensity training all of the time. Some athletes enjoy doing some moderately intense exercise during this training cycle and that is fine as long as it is controlled, done with purpose and makes up a lower portion of your entire training volume. Be sure that your longer duration training is spent in your aerobic training zone, as these sessions are what matter the most during this training cycle. Decades of research have proven that with aerobic training, the body becomes more efficient in using fat as fuel. This is the exact response you want during this time of your training year so pull back your reigns of going out too hard or too fast in this training cycle.

COMPETITION CYCLE METABOLIC EFFICIENCY PLANNING

Moving on to your next training cycle after your preparatory season brings different physical goals. From a metabolic efficiency standpoint, your main goal should now be to maintain and "protect" the benefits that you acquired during the preparatory cycle and reap the rewards of your hard work. Through personal testing on athletes, I have noticed that it can take as little as 2-3 weeks to see positive metabolic efficiency results when aerobic training is emphasized and nutrition periodization concepts, specifically following a more well-balanced daily macronutrient eating plan, are implemented. Interestingly, through my testing, I have found that it takes about the same amount of time to become metabolically inefficient when altering the nutrition plan (consuming too many carbohydrates and not enough lean protein and healthy fats). Therefore, it is extremely important to realize that you can lose all of the metabolic efficiency benefits from the previous cycle in as little as 2-3 weeks.

While it is a bit tricky to navigate this training cycle that is filled with higher intensity training, it is not impossible. The "ace in your pocket" is your daily nutrition plan. Keeping your macronutrients in balance during this higher intensity training is of utmost importance. Will you need more carbohydrates to fuel training? Sometimes yes, sometimes no. There are many factors behind periodizing your carbohydrate intake.

Much of the reason that you can revert back to being metabolically inefficient during your competitive season is because you will probably swap some of you aerobic training with more intense training. Additionally, you are likely to include more carbohydrate to fuel your workouts and use more during competition. Let's take a closer look at both of these and how you can make the most of your newly acquired metabolic efficiency throughout your competitive season.

NUTRITION STRATEGIES

The competition cycle is not normally the time to train in a chronic state of glycogen depletion. However, depending on when your competitions are scheduled and the nature of your training program design, it may be beneficial at times to introduce a short-term manipulation of your nutrition plan by training in a semi-depleted glycogen state. This is certainly not recommended long-term but can be beneficial during times of lighter training (in between competitions where a short transition or recovery will be taken) or even during an extended taper. I know it may seem a bit odd, mostly because you have not heard this concept before but please do not take this as a promotion of a low carbohydrate diet during your entire competitive season. Rather, I am encouraging you to maintain your nutrient balance, shift it accordingly based on your energy expenditure (by employing the concept of nutrition periodization) and not consume too high of carbohydrates when they are not needed. Far too many athletes justify an extremely high level of carbohydrate consumption because they are competing but remember, unless you have competitions every weekend or quality training sessions each day, you do not need consistently high stores of carbohydrate all of the time. Even if you do have frequent competitions, periodizing all of your macronutrient intake is the smartest thing you can do to promote good recovery strategies and to maintain competition body weight and composition.

This may be difficult for you to do but maintaining metabolic efficiency during the competitive season typically does not contain the term "carbohydrate loading". For athletes who become metabolically efficient, carbohydrate loading, in the true sense of the term, is simply not necessary. Slightly increasing carbohydrate intake in the window before and after a competition is justified but not at significantly high levels that are proposed in typical carbohydrate loading protocols. Maintaining nutrient balance throughout this training cycle without major shifts in any one nutrient will maintain the metabolic efficiency that you taught your body to have in your previous training cycle.

Sure, you may need to consume more carbohydrates during certain times of this training cycle when training volume and intensity justify it. When this is the case, increase your daily carbohydrate intake by introducing whole grains and healthier starches that are good sources of fiber, vitamins and minerals. Be sure to introduce them slowly throughout the day and not all in one feeding. In the previous training cycle, you relied mostly on fruits, vegetables, beans, nuts and dairy products to provide your body enough carbohydrates to sustain normal daily functions to support your lower training load. Since your training load will be increased, it may be necessary to gradually increase overall carbohydrate intake to provide higher muscle glycogen stores before and after quality training sessions. However, caution must be taken when doing this. Do not treat this like a light switch and immediately "flip the switch" to a high carbohydrate eating plan. Treat it more like a dimmer light switch where you gradually change the amount of carbohydrate intake in a controlled manner. Rest assured, if you treat it as an on/off switch, it will nullify your positive metabolic efficiency changes.

Unfortunately, I see many athletes making too drastic of a macronutrient shift during these times and the balance of lean protein, healthy fat, fruits and vegetables and whole grains is not maintained. More often than not, the shift for some athletes becomes eating a very high starchy carbohydrate diet flooded with white bagels, pasta and rice with very little contribution from the other nutrients.

There is obviously a very delicate balance that needs to be achieved with your daily and training nutrition during this cycle. If more carbohydrates are needed, it is easier to maintain this balance by using whole grains and healthier starches in a more strategic manner, specifically in the 24 hours before and 12 hours after quality training sessions or competitions. Research has shown that glycogen stores can be improved in the 24 hours before a competition by including more carbohydrates throughout the day. Additionally, the 12 hours following competition are important for glycogen replenishment. This is where my "24/12 rule" originates from and it is used with great success with athletes during their competition season. The basic premise is that 24 hours before a high quality workout or competition, you should add a few more servings of whole grains and healthier starches throughout the day to improve your glycogen stores. Then, after the session or competition, you continue this pattern for 12 hours. After the 12 hours following the training session or competition, return back to your normal metabolically efficient eating program emphasizing a well-balanced nutrient profile.

I know that this principle is slightly different than what

has existed for many years and I understand that it will take a paradigm shift for you to fully grasp this concept. However, let me explain why traditional sports nutrition messaging may not be the most viable option for all athletes throughout the entire training year. The most popular reason for athletes to eat larger quantities of calories and carbohydrates is because they think that their bodies require this large amount to sustain consistent energy levels throughout a certain duration or intensity of exercise. This usually turns out to be true because the athlete did not teach his body how to properly use his internal fat stores and thus preserve his carbohydrate stores in earlier season training. In simple terms, he did not follow a more balanced macronutrient eating plan and did not devote enough time to aerobic training when he should have. Because the body is using more carbohydrates, it needs more carbohydrates to sustain training. Therefore, he needs to eat more carbohydrates during training and competition in an effort to preserve his endogenous (internal) stores of carbohydrate and provide consistent energy to the working muscles and brain. This "old school" method may make sense at first, until you read farther into the story. Of course, I am going to provide that so be patient, it gets better!

Let's stop for a moment to review. If your goal is to preserve your endogenous carbohydrate stores, wouldn't it be easier to simply teach your body to rely more on using your endogenous fat stores throughout a variety of exercise intensities of training instead of constantly pumping your body with higher quantities of carbohydrates? Of course it makes sense and along with protecting these internal stores of carbohydrate, teaching your body to use more fat as fuel will also help to reduce the risk of GI distress, as I described earlier.

As a sport dietitian, a majority of the work I do with athletes is troubleshooting GI distress patterns and developing plans to minimize their negative impact on performance.

As an athlete, it is my top priority to avoid GI distress while I am training and competing. I am sure you feel the same way no matter what type of athlete you are or sport you participate in.

Of course there is another side to this and I have had the argument posed to me about trying to match energy intake and energy expenditure as closely as possible. That is, attempting to eat as much as the body can handle to try to minimize the energy deficit between calories burned and calories consumed during training or competition. While this may initially seem like a valid option, the logistics simply do not make sense and are not supported by what really happens in an athlete's body during competition. For example, if an athlete is estimated to expend 10,000 calories during a competition such as an Ironman triathlon with a projected finish time around 13 hours (this is a rough estimation of calorie expenditure for the sake of my example), how many calories could this athlete consume throughout this race? Eight-thousand? Five-thousand? Is there a correct answer? Unfortunately, the answer is not as easy as plugging some numbers into a calculation. Biology does not work that way.

Current sports nutrition research states that the body can "safely" absorb up to 90 grams (360 calories) of carbohydrate per hour. Assuming that all athletes could absorb up to this amount per hour (very few athletes can and in fact, the initial research was performed on male cyclists), approximately 4,680 calories in the form of carbohydrate could be consumed (360 calories multiplied by 13 hours). Protein contribution to energy intake and expenditure is minimal when carbohydrates are consumed so I will not factor that into the equation. In this example, this athlete could consume about 47% of the calories that are being expended. This is a very high and extremely generous estimate and is rarely seen in real life situations during competition where intensity is moderate to high. Of course there are some athletes who fall outside of the bell shaped curve and there always will be these exceptions. As stated previously, the normal range of energy intake that I have found in real-life is 15-35% of energy expenditure, depending on the competition type, duration and intensity.

Thus the question again arises, "if you cannot replace all of the energy that is being used during exercise, why not train your body to use more by eating more?" The next layer of this argument progresses to assume that you can preserve internal carbohydrate stores by eating more carbohydrates. This thought process is questionable because if you eat more carbohydrates, you will rely more on the ingested carbohydrates and thus you will need to feed greater quantities more often. You may minimize the use of glycogen stores but you still have to eat a large amount to obtain this state and this may lead to a higher risk of GI distress. However, as you have learned, this is the exact opposite feeding strategy that you are trying to accomplish when teaching your body to become more metabolically efficient.

This thought process of teaching the body to absorb more carbohydrates by eating more calories does not make practical sense. If you consume a higher carbohydrate food or meal on a consistent basis, you have a higher insulin response and this decreases the body's ability to oxidize fat along with the possibility of contributing to poor blood lipid (fat) management and a host of other health issues (as discussed in Chapter 2).

Additionally, let's look at this from a practical standpoint when you are competing. What if your sport requires you to be away from a central location where food and fluids are located? The food you need during competition may not be readily available which poses yet another problem of not being able to feed yourself the calories that you need. If you teach your body to need more carbohydrates per hour, you must have these available more frequently during competition. How will you carry these carbohydrates? Will the specific foods, beverages or products be available to you at and during your competition? The sport of ultra-running comes to mind. It is nearly impossible for these athletes to carry all of their required calories, especially if they need to feed themselves high quantities. Wouldn't it make more sense from a pure logistics standpoint to rely more on your internal fat stores to fuel a good portion of your competition so you do not have to carry as much fuel? Of course it would! Yet another reason to become and more importantly, remain metabolically efficient.

Maintaining metabolic efficiency during the competition cycle has obvious benefits for athletes exercising and competing longer than a few hours but it has just as much application for athletes who compete in shorter durations. Because intensity is greater during these shorter events. nutrients that are introduced to the body are not digested as easily. As you have read previously, the more opportunities you introduce calories to the body at higher intensities, the greater the risk for GI distress. Fewer feedings means a reduced chance of GI distress. I know many athletes from a host of different sports who make a concerted effort to minimize their hourly calorie intake as much as they can during competition so they maintain a "clean gut" and do not have to worry about having any digestive issues.

It is true that you need more carbohydrates at higher intensities of exercise. However, by improving your metabolic efficiency, you increase your ability to use more fat at higher intensities thus you will be able to use more fat throughout the exercise and decrease the use of carbohydrate until it is really needed. Of course, there is a caveat to this. You should not attempt to reduce your competition calorie and carbohydrate needs if you have not spent the time improving your metabolic efficiency. If you approach a competition without putting in the time to train your body to use more fat and you decrease your calorie intake, you will bonk, end of story. It will not be pretty.

You must treat metabolic efficiency as you do your training program. Both should be given adequate time to adapt and improve. You certainly cannot expect to have a stellar competition when you have only been training for a couple of weeks and the same is true with nutrition and metabolic efficiency.

An interesting observation I have made over the years when working with athletes who compete in shorter competitions is that the majority of the competition nutrition plan is focused on hydration and electrolyte use. Not much emphasis is placed on increasing the amount of calories consumed per hour. Will extra calories be needed in a shorter competition? Not as many as most athletes believe, especially if they have spent the time during their preparatory cycle improving their body's metabolic efficiency. I firmly believe that media influence has had a tremendous influence on athletes which teaches them to eat more during competitions. Using some basic biochemistry, digestion and exercise physiology principles along with conducting metabolic testing on athletes, I have been able to provide a more realistic, healthy way of preparing the body to compete that includes using a higher proportion of fat as fuel.

You have now heard the more popular arguments that I have received when teaching athletes and coaches the process of becoming more metabolically efficient. I can politely provide a rebuttal to these as you have read but in the end what really matters is what works best for you. My goal is to make you a better athlete, to experience less GI distress and succeed without nutrition being a limiter. I encourage each athlete I work with to become more metabolically efficient during their preparatory cycle and pay particular attention to how they feel during the day in respect to their energy levels and how their body responds during and after training sessions. Apply this same knowledge and skill set to your competition cycle and give this metabolic efficiency concept a chance. From a physiological and metabolic standpoint, it works, no question about it. But because our bodies change so often, you must adapt this to your individual nutrition and training programs to determine the true benefits.

Remember that I want to make you more metabolically efficient to need fewer calories per hour during training and competition. Whether it is 25 percent or 60 percent less than what you would usually consume does not matter. The point is that you are supplying more of your body's energy needs through stored fat and less by supplemental carbohydrates. Of course, by teaching your body to need less, you should start by consuming fewer calories per hour during training. It is always better to start with a lower amount of calories and add them gradually rather than start too high, overfeed your body and experience GI distress.

And yes, it is okay to introduce sports nutrition products to sustain performance but please use them responsibly. Remember, you have developed the ability to not rely as much on your internal carbohydrate stores so you do not need to over-consume drinks, bars, gels and chews. Use them as you need to but be smart about it. My Periodization Plates™ accounts for

Periodization Plates™

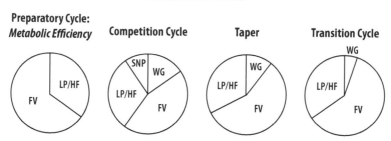

LP/HF: Lean Protein and Healthy Fats
FV: Fruits and Vegetables
WG: Whole Grains
SNP: Sports Nutrition Products

this but take note to the amount in your daily nutrition plan. Use real food as your primary fuel whenever possible.

TRAINING STRATEGIES

This is not a book about training design so I will not go into program development in great detail. However, in terms of metabolic efficiency, you learned earlier that aerobic exercise contributes to enhanced physiological adaptations in using fat as energy. The competition training cycle normally emphasizes higher intensity training to improve speed, power, economy and strength, all for good reason of improving performance. Many athletes have asked me if they lose their metabolic efficiency when they increase the intensity of their training. The not so simple answer is that it depends on how many training sessions are high intensity versus aerobic, where your metabolic efficiency point is located before entering this training cycle and of course, your daily macronutrient intake.

If you are consistently training at a higher intensity than your MEP, then your body will begin to oxidize more carbohydrates, that's basic energy system mechanics. However, the work you did earlier in the year to improve your metabolic efficiency will not be lost for the simple reason that all of your training sessions will not be at high intensities (at least they shouldn't be). All energy systems will be used and aerobic training will still be present even in this higher intensity training cycle.

However, there is another side to this story. I have witnessed many athletes complete their quality training sessions successfully at higher intensity but fail to meet their goals of staying aerobic during the lesser quality sessions where the primary objective of the workout is to remain aerobic. They seem to drift into the tempo and lower end threshold training zones during aerobic sessions. My recommendation to you, keeping metabolic efficiency in mind, is to put the quality work in when it is needed and prescribed in your training program but also respect your lower quality training sessions and recovery days and when these are on your schedule, fight the urge to increase the intensity. Stay aerobic and you will continue to support your body's improved metabolic efficiency.

There is one additional method to discuss that can assist with maintaining metabolic efficiency during the competition cycle. Completing aerobic focused training sessions in a lower glycogen state can assist the body in oxidizing fat but this practice can be tricky to implement as it can have a negative impact on the quality of your training and recovery if not done properly. If you would like to try this, do it only for aerobic training sessions lasting less than 3 hours. I recommend eating a good balance of carbohydrate, protein and fat prior to the workout then consuming only water and electrolytes throughout the training session. This will control your insulin level before training which will allow your body to oxidize fat more efficiently during training. After these types of sessions, it is extremely important to not overindulge and eat everything in sight. Remember, this is an aerobic training session. You should repeat your pre-workout feeding in the same manner by choosing a balance of carbohydrates, lean protein and healthy fat only if you are hungry or have a quality workout in the next 24 hours. Many athletes make a larger portion of a balanced meal or snack such as a fruit smoothie with a protein source (milk or whey protein isolate powder) and have half before the workout and the other half after the workout. It's an easy way to do it but what is important is for you to find what works best for your specific needs.

The take-home message is that it is not necessary to stop your higher intensity workouts. Rather, respect your lower intensity training sessions when they are on your schedule as these will be your metabolically efficient stabilizing exercise sessions.

TAPER NUTRITION

This section would not be complete without a few words about nutrition during a taper. This is by far one of the most confusing times of the year for athletes and their nutrition plan. Some athletes have challenges regulating their body weight during the taper due to the lower volume of training and lower energy expenditure. The concept of nutrition periodization has great efficacy during this time. Matching energy intake with energy expenditure is the goal throughout the entire year but it becomes especially important during a taper. Remember my "eat to train" mantra. When training load decreases, your nutrition plan should support that.

This will certainly not come as a surprise but one of the best ways to ensure weight stability during a taper is to focus on eating metabolically efficient, similar to the plan described for the preparatory training cycle with a few minor adjustments. Yes, you heard correctly. I do not support significantly altering the nutrition plan in terms of the macronutrient intake during a taper, even for athletes competing in longer durations. There could be a reduction in the quantity of food eaten depending on the planned decrease in training volume but be sure to remain in macronutrient balance as I have described throughout this book. You have spent a good portion of your nutrition training with the focus on improving metabolic efficiency and the worst thing you can do is eat in the exact opposite manner during your taper. Depending on how long your taper lasts, you can negate the benefits you worked so hard at developing by throwing your nutrition in the trash and creating imbalance in your daily nutrient intake.

Specifically, I am referring to carbohydrate loading. Remember the story behind high carbohydrate intake, the insulin response and fat oxidation? If you have followed a metabolically efficient daily nutrition plan up to this point, there is no need to

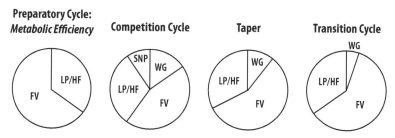

Periodization Plates™

LP/HF: Lean Protein and Healthy Fats
FV: Fruits and Vegetables
WG: Whole Grains
SNP: Sports Nutrition Products

introduce a traditional carbohydrate loading regimen the days leading up to competition. In fact, there may be no reason for sports nutrition products such as energy bars and drinks until competition day (I actually recommend this whenever possible). The message is simple: remain in nutrient balance by eating lean protein, healthy fats, fruits and vegetables and whole grains (if you are including those) and you will successfully navigate your way through your taper, ready for competition day. I have even had athletes who have been successful in maintaining body weight and energy without including any form of whole grain during their taper. Refer to my Periodization Plates™ as a guide to nutrient partitioning during the taper.

TRANSITION CYCLE (ALSO CALLED THE OFF-SEASON) METABOLIC EFFICIENCY PLANNING

This training cycle poses the most challenges for athletes for many reasons. You are likely used to consuming sports nutrition products such as sports drinks, energy bars, gels and other products to sustain your nutrition needs during your competition cycle. You will not need these now (trust me, you do not) but one of the most difficult things for you to do is to flip the behavior change switch and convince your body to stop using them. It's a habit and one that you have probably fine-tuned in the past few months during your competition cycle. While there is certainly nothing wrong with using these products during the right time of the competition year, remember that they are formulated for a specific reason and it is not to supply your body with extra calories during your off-season. Using these products will simply add to unnecessary increases in body weight and body fat. Stop using them. Place them in a box, tape it up like you are shipping it across the country and hide it in a place where it cannot be easily found such as a garage, basement or attic. Out of sight, out of mind.

Your second challenge is the holidays. Because this time of the year falls during the holiday season for some athletes, it is worth mentioning. I know it may be difficult to navigate the social pressures, parties and bountiful offerings of food that are found at social engagements but one of the best things you can do, while remembering to eat for enhanced metabolic efficiency, is to limit your nutritional "misses". These "misses" are any food or beverage such as chocolate, pastries and alcohol that you cannot classify into the lean protein, healthy fat, fruit, vegetable or whole grain categories. I know it sounds easy on paper but it is more difficult than you think. This will require some planning, preparation and a bit of will power since it is a change in habit.

Lastly, let us not forget that one of the main objectives of this training cycle, if in fact you are taking an off-season, is to have fun without much training program structure. This is difficult to manage for most athletes because they are used to following a very regimented training program with frequent competitions. Now, all of a sudden, you stop this type of training and your self-confidence can be affected. Depression and guilty feelings sparked by a lower training load may also enter the picture. Allow yourself to have a mental and physical break and enjoy it. You only come about this training cycle once a year and it is normally very short. Don't waste your time and energy stressing about your fitness level. Your nutrition plan will support your reduced energy expenditure.

NUTRITION STRATEGIES

Your primary goal during the transition cycle is to regain your foundational metabolic efficiency. It took a bit of a "hit" during your competition season due to the higher intensity training and altered nutrition plan but it won't take long to get it back to normal. It is important to periodize your nutrition now to use your metabolic systems to improve your efficiency. This can be easily done by using the nutrition strategies I presented in the preparatory cycle section with a few minor changes. I will again refer you to my Periodization Plates™ as a guide.

First, because this is the time of the year when one of your main goals should be having fun without much structure, allow yourself the flexibility of eating a variety of foods without hav-

Periodization Plates™

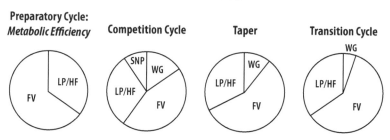

Preparatory Cycle:
Metabolic Efficiency Competition Cycle Taper Transition Cycle

LP/HF: Lean Protein and Healthy Fats
FV: Fruits and Vegetables
WG: Whole Grains
SNP: Sports Nutrition Products

ing to count or restrict calories or follow a "diet". In fact, those rarely work anyway but that is a topic of another book.

Place your attention on including predominantly lean protein, healthy fat (with an emphasis on omega-3 fat) and fruits and vegetables as your daily staple foods. Increase your daily protein intake during this cycle as it will improve your feeling of fullness which will control your hunger response much better. This will help you control your body weight and body composition with more success. Minimize and limit your whole grain and starch intake as much as possible. You will receive the nutrients your body needs from other foods. I know it will be tough with all of the holiday goodies that challenge you but do your best. Your body prefers being metabolically efficient much more than the opposite but you do have to allow yourself to be human every so often and enjoy life's nutritional pleasures. Savor them in small amounts. Enjoy the taste and texture of these "misses" and it should prevent you from over-consuming them. I use the word "should" on purpose. Put in a good effort and keep in mind that emotions usually drive food choices during the off-season. Manage your emotions and the "why" behind your eating patterns. Most athletes will overeat due to higher stress, boredom or even social pressures. Knowing your triggers can help you navigate your off-season eating with much more ease and success.

It is almost certain that you were used to a slightly higher daily and training calorie intake to maintain and replenish your glycogen stores during your competition cycle. However, during the transition cycle, a high calorie load is not necessary. In fact, it can be extremely detrimental. This is much easier said than done because moving from a higher to a lower calorie intake requires a behavior change rather than the "I will do this tomorrow" approach. It would be nice if it were that easy but it is not for most athletes due to the complexity of the behavior change process. Allow yourself a little time to scale down your total calorie load and re-focus your nutritional sights with the nutrition recommendations I made in the previous paragraph. Don't forget to get all of your sports nutrition supplements out of sight and out of mind. This simple yet effective strategy will allow you to return to a high metabolically efficient state again.

Lastly, it is important to remember to feed your body based on biological hunger instead of habitual hunger. An example of the latter includes using your watch as your meal-time guide as you were likely accustomed to in your competition cycle. Listen to your biological hunger cues, feed your body the appropriate nutrients by using my Periodization Plates™ and feel your fullness. Trust your instincts and don't use certain time intervals to tell you when you are hungry.

EXERCISE STRATEGIES

If you allow your body to do one thing during this cycle it should be to learn the difference between training and exercising. This is the most important point you can emphasize as you move from your competition season to your off-season. Let me explain this further. During this cycle most athletes take a couple of weeks to a couple of months of down time from their primary sport to rejuvenate their bodies and minds. This is a very necessary component of sport and well-deserved after coming off of a long competition season. If you continue to follow a structured training program, as you have been the last 8-11 months, then you are not in an off-season. However, if you are not formally training (defined as following a structured program) and simply exercising to maintain fitness and have fun, your nutritional goals become much easier to implement because they do not become a chore. You do not have to worry about supplying your body enough energy to sustain training because you are not training.

One of the best things you can do to improve metabolic efficiency is to reduce the intensity of your exercise and focus on aerobic exercise once again. I usually do not promote the use of heart rate monitors or other pieces of technology as monitoring devices during this time of the year. Use subjective measures such as your breathing and rating of perceived exertion as cues and by all means, have fun. These combined will almost ensure that you are remaining at lower intensities during exercise. As you now know, staying mostly aerobic will induce metabolic and cellular changes that will improve your body's ability to use its stored nutrients, specifically fat. Make the mental switch from "training" to "exercising", focus on aerobic activity and try new ways to get the heart pumping.

Chapter 6
Case Studies

The following case studies will give you an idea of the impact of nutrition and exercise on metabolic efficiency. I provide three distinct athlete scenarios with different analyses so you can further your understanding of this topic and more importantly, see how I bring the concept to life with real athletes. These will hopefully provide you a few "a-ha moments" and ones that you can implement in your own training and nutrition programs.

CASE STUDY #1

THE METABOLICALLY INEFFICIENT RUNNER

This first case study is of a 35 year-old male, recreational long-distance runner who was at the end of his transition cycle and entering his preparatory cycle of training. He was training for his first ultra-endurance running race of 100 miles and wanted to be sure that he could fuel himself during this longer race without having nutritional or GI issues.

He had traditionally used many sports nutrition products such as sports drinks, energy bars and gels in previous training years and competitions and found that as he competed in any race longer than a marathon, his stomach would begin to have problems and he would get GI distress. My first order of business was to assess his current state of metabolic efficiency.

The graph below depicts his metabolic assessment which shows a high degree of metabolic inefficiency. He was tested running on a treadmill at different paces after an adequate twenty minute warm-up. This was an incremental test with the speed of the treadmill increasing every five minutes and the incline held at 1% throughout. He was breathing into a mouthpiece connected to a metabolic cart so that his oxygen and carbon dioxide could be analyzed.

As can be seen, a large amount of carbohydrates were being used from the beginning of exercise and he was very inefficient at oxidizing fat, even at lower intensities. Obviously, this is not an ideal scenario for his ultra-running goals since he would have to consume more supplemental carbohydrates because he oxidizes a higher amount and this could increase his risk of GI distress. The metabolic assessment was invaluable because we were able to get a clear picture of what his body was doing on the inside and what interventions needed to be made from the outside.

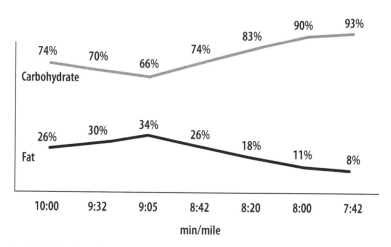

First metabolic test on ultra-endurance runner.

As you can see from the graph showing his second metabolic assessment performed three months later, the benefits he had shown with our intervention were significant. During these three months of preparatory training, he decreased his total daily carbohydrate intake from 7.7 grams to 5.4 grams per kilogram of body weight (almost all from reducing whole grain and starch intake) and increased his lean protein and healthy fat consumption. He also used a heart rate monitor to train more effectively in his aerobic training zones without temptations of veering into his higher intensity zones.

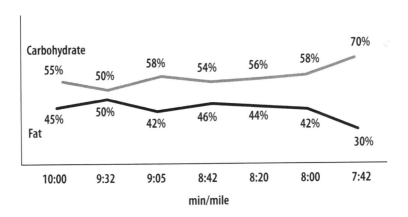

Follow-up metabolic test on ultra-endurance runner at month three.

As can been seen, he improved his macronutrient partitioning to favor using fat as fuel as the intensity of exercise increased. This change had a significant impact on his nutritional needs during training. He trained his body to rely more on internal fat stores and preserve his internal carbohydrates stores thus he did not have to try to feed himself as many carbohydrates per hour during training as he had in the past. In fact, he reported to normally consume about 250-300 calories per hour before our intervention and afterwards, he trained his body to consume 100-150 calories per hour with no decrease in performance. Aerobic runs and threshold/intensity runs were all sustained at 100-150 calories per hour. His incidence of GI distress was gone and he felt like he had a much more consistent energy level throughout the day and during training.

During his longer training runs, he would consume mostly water, electrolyte supplements, peanut butter and jelly sandwiches and cheese sandwiches. For any run under 3 hours, he focused mostly on using water and electrolytes if needed as dictated by environmental conditions. He made sure to have a balanced snack consisting of lean protein, healthy fat and a fruit in the hour before his training.

Interestingly, he shifted from using a great deal of sports nutrition products to using more whole foods and he found it worked much better for him since it provided less simple sugars. This also provided him more of a "clean gut" which kept his GI distress symptoms at bay. Because he was training for such a long competition, reducing his hourly calorie needs was of extreme benefit for the reasons previously discussed in addition to decreasing the added weight from food that he had to carry with him during his training.

Following his progress throughout his competition, we realized that with this small but significant metabolic change, he decreased his calories per hour needs during training by 50% with a performance improvement of over 1 hour during his 100-mile trail running race. Surprisingly, he averaged 133 calories per hour over the course of his 100-mile race and set a new personal record at the same time!

CASE STUDY #2:

ELITE MOUNTAIN BIKER WHO BONKS FREQUENTLY

This second case study is of an elite, male mountain biker who was having significant challenges feeding himself during races which led to many sub-par finishes caused by an energy deficit. He could not afford to take his hands off his handlebars long enough to eat due to the high level of competition and his normal placement in the front pack. This was leading him to becoming malnourished in his longer races which caused him very poor placing overall. I looked at his overall daily nutrition plan and there were a few tweaks I could have made to it but I knew that they would not be enough to provide him what he needed for his races that lasted three or more hours. Thus, I wanted to make him more efficient in using the nutrients he already had stored in his body.

He came to me with a short time in between his competitive season and his preparatory cycle and wanted to make the largest impact he could on his body's ability to use nutrients. I discussed the metabolic efficiency concept with him and he agreed to take the challenge of improving his efficiency. Reducing his reliance on supplemental carbohydrates during the race was a key goal for us since logistically, he could not consume what he needed.

Because he had just finished his race season and was coming off of a very high intensity race block with a very small emphasis on aerobic training, I began to paint the picture in my head of what his MEP would look like (it wasn't pretty!). We then discussed his eating program and as I expected, he followed a very high carbohydrate diet with little emphasis on protein and fat. He justified eating this way because he was racing. The picture became even more clear because as I described previously, eating a high carbohydrate diet will lead to a higher oxidation of carbohydrates. Thus, I had a suspicion that he would not have a MEP and that he would be extremely metabolically inefficient.

I was correct as can be seen from his metabolic assessment below. He did not have a MEP and as I learned, his normal average power output during races normally exceeded 250 watts. It was clear from the metabolic assessment that his body relied largely on carbohydrates to fuel his energy needs. It is no wonder that he told me that he either bonked or felt very low energy towards the last loop or few miles of his races. He wasn't able to feed his body enough carbohydrates due to his inability in using his internal fat stores.

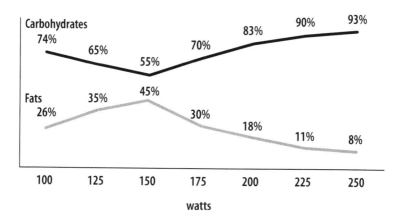

First metabolic assessment on elite mountain biker.

After we discussed the interpretation of his first metabolic assessment and knowing that he only had three weeks to make changes due to his short transition cycle, we set forth on a somewhat aggressive training and nutrition plan. I termed it aggressive from the standpoint that he would follow the plan with very few deviations. He agreed to this even though the three weeks spanned the holidays and he would be at his parents home the entire time. He was very motivated but I had to inform him that I had never tested the effects of aerobic training and nutrition on metabolic efficiency in as little as three weeks so the timeframe of making a positive impact on his metabolic efficiency would be a bit of an experiment. We were both ready as we were eager to see the changes. Even a small impact would yield positive results.

His exercise plan for the three weeks consisted of 100% aerobic training-no tempo, no threshold, only aerobic. His program consisted of snowshoeing and cross-country skiing with no cycling. He made sure he would stay in his aerobic intensity zones by monitoring his heart rate. He had a recently performed a lactate threshold test and knew what heart rates corresponded to aerobic training.

I informed him that he was not in a training cycle and that his psychological focus needed to be on being a person who exercised rather than an athlete who trained. This helped him tremendously as he was able to step out of his typical athlete lifestyle that usually includes hard training and a very high carbohydrate diet. Once he was able to establish his new role for the next three weeks, I structured his eating program to reflect this lower volume and intensity training load which included eating primarily lean protein, healthy fats and fruits and vegetables. Whole grains and starches were minimized and only eaten when absolutely necessary.

As you can see, I am not a fan of prescribing calories or having athletes count calories. I believe in a much more simplistic approach that allows athletes to be empowered and educate themselves by learning more about their body, their hunger cues and biological versus habitual versus emotional hunger.

With this simple nutrition plan, I was able to almost ensure his ability to comply because it was not numbers based nor did he have to count calories. He appreciated that greatly.

Of course he did enjoy the occasional holiday treat but he kept that under control without bingeing. When he returned from his short break, we did another metabolic efficiency assessment and I was pleasantly surprised, even somewhat shocked. I didn't know what to expect since I had not implemented nor quantified a metabolic efficiency plan in such a small window of time but as you can see from the graph below, the assessment at week three was a huge success and spoke volumes regarding the body's ability to make a metabolic shift in a short amount of time.

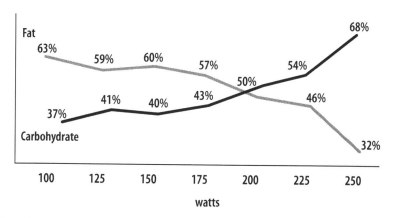

Second metabolic assessment done 3 weeks after nutrition and exercise intervention on elite mountain biker.

He achieved a MEP in only 3 weeks. This had shown that a short-term exercise and nutrition intervention can indeed have a significant impact on metabolic efficiency and the ability to teach the body to use more internal fat stores for energy. This allowed him to race better because his body was not relying as much on carbohydrates during his races. He found that he had much more energy during his races. We also ensured that he had a balance of carbohydrate, lean protein and healthy fat in his pre-race meal to balance blood sugar and insulin levels rather than rely on his past sports nutrition regimen which contained mostly simple carbohydrates in the sixty-minute window prior to competition.

CASE STUDY #3:

RECREATIONAL ATHLETE SEEKING WEIGHT LOSS

This last case study is of a 50 year-old male, recreational tri-athlete who was seeking weight and body fat loss to improve performance. His main focus for his upcoming competition season was to compete in a half-Ironman and set a new personal record. I began working with him in November and his main competition was in June the following year.

He voluntarily logged his food frequently which allowed me to analyze his nutrient intake based on his body weight and take a close look at his progression of nutrient intake to his feelings of fullness, weight loss, performance and recovery. In essence, I was able to compare quantitative with qualitative measures and feedback. While I did not have metabolic assessment data from my personal testing, I was able to use his food and exercise logging to provide a quantitative analysis based on macronutrient shifting. He had metabolic testing done at his facility and the trends of his RER were extremely positive throughout this process. In the beginning, his exercise RER showed that he was oxidizing a high amount of carbohydrate and as we progressed and implemented a macronutrient shifting plan, his RER decreased during exercise reflecting an increase in fat oxidation.

The following graph compares his daily carbohydrate, protein and fat intake in grams per kilogram of body weight (g/kg) throughout the months. In November of 2008, his carbohydrate intake was higher than his protein and fat intake. This is typical but interestingly, his carbohydrate intake was

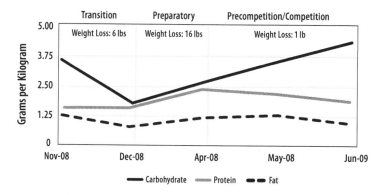

Graph showing the trend of the quantity of carbohydrate, protein and fat intake throughout the months for recreational triathlete.

only 3.5 g/kg, which is on the lower end of the published data that describes athletes daily carbohydrate needs. His protein intake was 1.5 g/kg and fat was 1.1 g/kg, both in the scientific research ranges.

Because he wanted to lose weight, I knew I would need to manipulate his macronutrients to favor a metabolic shift. His training was moderate to low in volume since he was entering his transition cycle thus I asked him to reduce his carbohydrate and fat intake as the first steps in this journey. As shown in the graph above, in December of 2008, his carbohydrate intake was 1.7 g/kg, protein intake remained the same at 1.5 g/kg and fat intake decreased to 0.7 g/kg. The trend for weight loss was positive but I knew that we also had to manipulate his protein intake so that was my next order of business.

He wanted to lose more weight than the six pounds he had seen in November and December but he was also beginning his preparatory cycle in January so we had to negotiate feeding him enough so he could still sustain his training. Because his training was mostly aerobic, I knew the opportunity was perfect to introduce another macronutrient "shift" as it would not have a negative impact on his performance. The next intervention included increasing his daily protein consumption and a slight increase in carbohydrate to move him closer to the lower range of carbohydrate intake found in published literature (3 g/kg). This would support his increased energy expenditure needs as he began training again.

From late December/early January to April, he changed his daily nutrition habits so that he consumed 2.6 g/kg of carbohydrate (up from 1.7g/kg in the previous cycle) and protein increased to 2.3 g/kg (up from 1.5 g/kg). Fat intake did slightly increase to 1.1 g/kg but this was not as significant as the other nutrient changes.

By shifting his protein intake higher and keeping his carbohydrate and fat intake under control at somewhat lower levels, we were able to induce a more successful rate of weight loss. His energy expenditure was increased due to his training load but because he was still in his preparatory training cycle, he was not burning an extremely high amount of calories. The interaction of his aerobic exercise and macronutrient shift, which included the increase in protein as the primary change, allowed his body to lose another 16 pounds in 2.5 months. This was exactly what he had hoped for to assist him with improving his performance in his upcoming competition.

We were most successful at reducing his body weight during his preparatory training cycle which allowed him to enter his pre-competition cycle lighter. Because his training intensity and energy expenditure would be increased in April and May, I did not want weight loss to be his primary focus during that stage. Rather, I wanted him to make the shift to performance. To do this, he increased his carbohydrate intake from 2.6 g/kg to 3.5 g/kg, decreased his protein intake from 2.3 g/kg to 2.1 g/kg and increased his fat intake from 1.1 g/kg to 1.2 g/kg. As you can see from the weight trends graph below, there was a slight decrease (1 pound) in his weight from April to May but because he was seeing very good performance adaptations during training, our plan was to halt his weight loss and focus on performance markers only.

An interesting observation that he made and that has been confirmed by other athletes whom I have worked with on improving metabolic efficiency was that he was not as hungry after quality training sessions. In the past, when he was eating too many carbohydrates relative to his energy expenditure, he felt ravenous and craved sugar after long duration and high intensity workouts. He did not experience that now which helped maintain his blood sugar and thus his weight stability as can be seen from the graph below.

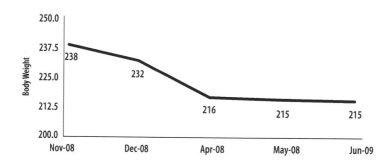

Graph showing the athlete's body weight trends throughout the months.

Moving into his competition training cycle in June, we shifted his nutrient intake once again (displaying the importance of periodizing nutrition to match physical training needs). His carbohydrate intake increased from 3.5 g/kg to 4.3 g/kg, protein decreased from 2.1 g/kg to 1.8 g/kg and fat decreased from 1.2 g/kg to 0.9 g/kg. This allowed him to maintain his fitness while supplying enough energy to support his performance as he approached his competition.

Over a period of just under 7 months, he made huge

strides in improving his metabolic efficiency through the manipulation of his daily nutrition coupled with his training load changes. This allowed him to rely less on supplemental carbohydrates during training and when he put his nutrition to the test during his race, it proved even more successful than we had thought.

The benefits that we saw really became obvious during his competition. During his half Ironman race in June, his average calorie intake was only 172 calories per hour with 29 grams coming from carbohydrate. Keep in mind that he competed at 215 pounds. At that body size, these hourly calories and grams of carbohydrate normally would not have come close to sustaining his energy needs. However, by shifting his internal energy stores and enabling him to use more fat as fuel at higher intensities, he was able to set a new personal record by 25 minutes, all while consuming less calories than he ever had before! And the best part was that he had no incidence of GI distress!

Parting Thoughts

Improving metabolic efficiency works. I have more and more athletes proving this as their competitions come and go. The real key to being successful with metabolic efficiency is to check your preconceived notions of how you used to do things at the door. There is nothing crazy about what I am proposing. No unrealistic diet or fast or cleanse. It is merely incorporating known exercise physiology research and principles with the relatively new concept of nutrition periodization and macronutrient shifting.

Once you are ready to become more metabolically efficient, it will happen. But remember, you are changing the way you eat and your approach to training, both at the same time in some instances. Please do not expect your body to adapt overnight. These are behavior changes that I am proposing and they will take weeks to months to implement depending on your readiness to change. Be patient with yourself and perhaps start by implementing just a few of my concepts at a time instead of the entire thing all at once. Assess where you are in your readiness to change, your personality and what training cycle you are in before you embark upon this journey. You will be rewarded. It's just a matter of time!

Alas, this book is finally near the end and I thought I would leave you with some key take-home messages:

MESSAGE #1

Adopt a nutritional paradigm shift. As you approach your daily food selection, prioritize your feedings. If your training volume and intensity are low, you can easily fuel your body with lean protein, healthy fats, fruits and vegetables with the sporadic introduction of a whole grain or healthier starch if needed (or wanted). Give yourself time to ease into this to ensure that you will be successful. I have noticed that a 3-5 day "break-in" period is required followed by an implementation phase of about 3 weeks to really allow the new change to take effect. Use my Periodization Plates™ as a guide. A good rule of thumb is that when choosing food, first on your plate should be a source of lean protein and healthy, omega-3 rich fat, followed by a healthy portion of fruits and/or vegetables. If your training cycle demands it, save a little room for whole grains and healthier starches. Following this approach will ensure that you are consuming the necessary nutrients and quantities that will help promote metabolic efficiency. Remember, there is no need to count calories or measure serving sizes. By choosing your foods as I have suggested, your fullness factor will increase if you listen to your body and its hunger cues and feelings of satisfaction.

MESSAGE #2

Use the "out of sight, out of mind" thought process. Nutrition supplements such as sports drinks, energy bars and gels will inhibit your progress of reaching metabolic efficiency when used inappropriately during the wrong times of your training year. Focus on having well-balanced feedings as I have described in frequent intervals and save the nutrition supplements for your more intense training sessions and competitions. Remember, your goal is to teach your body to use its fat stores more efficiently and improper use of these products will hinder your progress.

MESSAGE #3

Most importantly, have fun with your nutrition and don't make it a chore. You don't have to count calories or measure your food. Simply shift your nutrients to match your specific training and metabolic goals throughout the year. Become proficient in the concept of nutrition periodization and implement it just as you do your training program.

The impact of a nutrition only intervention on the metabolic efficiency point is not entirely known and it is important to remember that it has not been scientifically scrutinized. However, proper nutrition planning, in addition to well-planned aerobic training throughout your training year, can likely have a more profound effect on the cellular adaptations versus only one of the variables by itself. The research on the nutrition part independently has just not been done yet in the manner that is applicable to athletes.

Through personal testing, I have begun to answer the question, "how long does it take to become metabolically inefficient". The answer thus far is just as quickly as it is developed, depending on the level of nutrition and exercise intervention. Thus, it becomes crucial to follow a properly periodized nutrition program year-round in order to teach the body to become more metabolically efficient in the early part of the preparatory cycle, then maintain it throughout the year by not switching to a super high carbohydrate eating plan. Maintain your macronutrient balance and you will remain metabolically efficient. Add whole grains and healthier starches when energy expenditure is high and too great to be satisfied from the carbohydrates supplied by fruits, vegetables, beans, nuts and dairy products.

I am just asking you to be smart with your nutrient selection and alter it throughout the year based on your training and metabolic efficiency goals.

As I am sure you have been able to determine from reading this book, metabolic efficiency can benefit your health and performance. Improving metabolic efficiency should be the primary goal in the early part of your training year and nutrition periodization should be implemented year-round in an effort to support your physical goals of each training cycle to improve and maintain metabolic efficiency. Adhere to the concepts I have presented throughout this book and you will be better able to use your internal fat stores for energy during training and competition while depending less on supplemental carbohydrates. In the end, you will be healthier due to a more balanced macronutrient intake which will spill over onto your performance.

The research behind this aspect of sports nutrition and exercise performance is still in its infancy and there are many exciting things to be learned throughout this journey. Thank you for your interest in this topic and for reading this book!

References and
Recommended Readings

1. Achten, J, Gleeson, M and Jeukendrup, AE. Determination of the exercise intensity that elicits maximal fat oxidation. Med Sci Sports Exerc 34: 92-97. 2002.

2. Achten, J and Jeukendrup, A. Maximal fat oxidation during exercise in trained men. Int J Sports Med 24: 603-608. 2003.

3. Achten, J and Jeukendrup, A. Relation between plasma lactate concentration and fat oxidation rates over a wide range of exercise intensities. Int J Sports Med 25: 32-37. 2004.

4. Achten, J and Jeukendrup, A. Optimizing fat oxidation through exercise and diet. Nutr 20: 716-727. 2004.

5. Bergman, BC and Brooks, GA. Respiratory gas-exchange ratios during graded exercise in fed and fasted trained and untrained men. J Appl Physiol 86: 479-487. 1999.

6. Brooks, GA. Mammalian fuel utilization during sustained exercise. Comp Biochem Physiol B Biochem Mol Biol 120: 89-107. 1998.

7. Brooks, GA and Mercier, J. Balance of carbohydrate and lipid utilization during exercise: the "crossover" concept. J Appl Physiol 76: 2253-2261. 1994.

8. Brooks, GA and Trimmer, JK. Glucose kinetics during high-intensity exercise and the crossover concept. J Appl Physiol 80: 1073-1075. 1996.

9. Carter, SL, Rennie, C and Tarnopolsky, MA. Substrate utilization duringendurance exercise in men and women after endurance training. Am J Physiol Endocrinol Metab 280: E898-907. 2001.

10. Coggan, AR, Raguso, CA, Gastaldelli, A, Sidossis, LS and Yeckel, CW. Fat metabolism during high-intensity exercise in endurance-trained and untrained men. Metabolism 49: 122-128. 2000.

11. Costill, DL, Fink, WJ, Getchell, LH, Ivy, JL and Witzmann, FA. Lipid metabolism in skeletal muscle of endurance-trained males and females. J Appl Physiol 47: 787-791. 1979.

12. Coyle, EF, Jeukendrup, AE, Oseto, MC, Hodgkinson, BJ and Zderic, TW. Low-fat diet alters intramuscular substrates and reduces lipolysis and fat oxidation during exercise. Am J Physiol Endocrinol Metab 280: E391-398. 2001.

13. Fattor, JA, Miller, BF, Jacobs, KA and Brooks, GA. Catecholamine response is attenuated during moderate intensity exercise in response to the lactate clamp. Am J Physiol Endocrinol Metab 288: E143-E147, 2005.

14. Fleming, J, Sharman, MJ, Avery, NG, Love, DM, Gomez, AL, Scheet, TP, Kraemer, WJ and Volek, JS. Endurance capacity and high-intensity exercise performance responses to a high-fat diet. Int J Sp Nutr Exerc Metab 13: 466-478. 2003.

15. Friedlander, AL, Casazza, GA, Horning, MA, Buddinger, TF and Brooks, GA. Effects of exercise intensity and training on lipid metabolism in young women. Am J Physiol 275: E853-863. 1998.

16. Friedlander, AL, Casazza, GA, Horning, MA, Huie, MJ, Piacentini, MF, Trimmer, JK and Brooks, GA. Training-induced alterations of carbohydrate metabolism in women: women respond differently from men. J Appl Physiol 85: 1175-1186. 1998.

17. Friedlander,, AL, Jacobs, KA, Fattor, JA, Horning, MA, Hagobian, TA, Bauer, TA, Wolfel, EE and Brooks, GA. Contributions of working muscle to whole body lipid metabolism vary with exercise intensity and training. Am J Physiol Endocrinol Metab. 292: E107-E116. 2007.

18. Goedecke, JH, St Clair Gibson, A, Grobler, L, Collins, M, Noakes, TD and Lambert, EV. Determinants of the variability in respiratory exchange ratio at rest and during exercise in trained athletes. Am J Physiol Endocrinol Metab 279: E1325-1334. 2000.

19. Helge, JW. Long-term fat diet adaptation effects on performance, training capacity, and fat utilization. Med Sci Sports Exerc 34(9): 1499-1504. 2002.

20. Helge, JW, Watt, PW, Richter, EA, Rennie, MJ and Kiens, B. Fat utilization during exercise: adaptation to a fat-rich diet increases utilization of plasma fatty acids and very low density lipoprotein-triacylglycerol in humans. J Physiol 537: 1009-1020. 2001.

21. Helge, JW, Wulff, B and Kiens, B. Impact of a fat-rich diet on endurance in man: role of the dietary period. Med Sci Sports Exerc 30(3): 456-461. 1998.

22. Horowitz, JF, Mora-Rodriguez, R, Byerley, LO and Coyle, EF. Lipolytic suppression following carbohydrate ingestion limits fat oxidation during exercise. Am J Physiol 273: E768-775. 1997.

23. Horton, TJ, Pagliassotti, MJ, Hobbs, K and Hill, JO. Fuel metabolism in men and women during and after long-duration exercise. J Appl Physiol 85: 1823-1832. 1998.

24. Jacobs, KA, Krauss, RM, Fattor, JA, Horning, MA, Friedlander, AL, Bauer, TA, Hagobian, TA, Wolfel, EE and Brooks, GA. Endurance training has little effect on active muscle fatty acid, lipoprotein, or triglyceride net balances. Am J Physiol Endocrinol Metab. 29: E656-665. 2006.

25. Jacobs, KA, Paul, DR, Deor, RJ, Hinchcliff, KW and Sherman, WM. Dietary composition influences short-term endurance training induced adaptations of substrate partitioning during exercise. Int J Sports Nutr Exerc Metab 14: 38-61. 2004.

26. Jeukendrup, AE. Regulation of fat metabolism in skeletal muscle. Ann NY Acad Sci 967: 217-235. 2002.

27. Klein, S, Coyle, EF and Wolfe, RR. Fat metabolism during low-intensity exercise in endurance-trained and untrained men. Am J Physiol 267: E934-940. 1994.

28. Kuo, CC, Fattor, JA, Henderson, GC and Brooks, GA. Effect of exercise intensity on lipid oxidation in fit young adults during exercise recovery. J Appl Physiol 99: 349-356. 2005.

29. Lambert, EV, Hawley, JA, Goedecke, J, Noakes, TD and Dennis, SC. Nutritional strategies for promoting fat utilization and delaying the onset of fatigue during pro-longed exercise. J Sport Sci 15: 315-324. 1997.

30. Lambert, EV, Speechly, DP, Dennis, SC and Noakes, TD. Enhanced endurance in trained cyclists during moderate intensity exercise following 2 weeks adaptation to a high fat diet. J Appl Physiol 69: 287-293. 1994.

31. Phillips, SM, Green, HJ, Tarnopolsky, MA, Heigenhauser, GF, Hill, RE and Grant, SM. Effects of training duration on substrate turnover and oxidation during exercise. J Appl Physiol 81: 2182-2191. 1996.

32. Romijn, JA, Coyle, EF, Sidossis, LS, Rosenblatt, J and Wolfe, RR. Substrate metabo-lism during different exercise intensities in endurance-trained women. J Appl Physiol 88: 1707-1714. 2000.

33. Sidossis, LS, Gastaldelli, A, Klein, S and Wolfe, RR. Regulation of plasma fatty acid oxidation during low- and high-intensity exercise. Am J Physiol 272: E1065-1070. 1997.

34. Spriet, LL. Regulation of skeletal muscle fat oxidation during exercise in humans. Med Sci Sports Exerc 34: 1477-1484. 2002.

35. Tarnopolsky, LJ, MacDougall, JD, Atkinson, SA, Tarnopolsky, MA and Sutton, JR. Gender differences in substrate for endurance exercise. J Appl Physiol 68: 302- 308. 1990.

36. Thompson, DL, Townsend, KM, Boughey, R, Patterson, K and Bassett, DR, Jr. Sub-strate use during and following moderate- and low-intensity exercise: implications for weight control. Eur J Appl Physiol Occup Physiol 78: 43-49. 1998.

About the Author

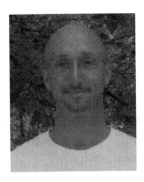 Bob Seebohar has worn many hats throughout his career. Starting out as an exercise physiologist by studying exercise and sports science in his undergraduate work, he turned to the fitness world upon exiting college but soon found himself asking more questions than he could answer so he decided to return to graduate school to expand his knowledge base. He received his first graduate degree in health and exercise science that had a large emphasis on metabolism and it was during this time where he was formally introduced to sports nutrition. Throughout graduate school, Bob worked with collegiate athletes, assisting them in improving their health and performance through nutrition and it was then that he realized that he had discovered his true passion of combining exercise with nutrition.

This led Bob to staying an extra year in graduate school to receive a second graduate degree in food science and human nutrition, mostly to satisfy the qualifications of becoming a Registered Dietitian (RD). He knew he would require that expertise to continue his work with athletes. After graduate school, Bob was extremely focused on becoming one of the best sport dietitians in the country and outlined a specific plan to attain this goal. Throughout the past 16 years, he has acquired valuable hands-on experience working with athletes of all ages and abilities and has fine tuned his approach to sports nutrition.

He has worked in the collegiate sports nutrition setting as a consultant to Colorado State University and the University of Northern Colorado, has held the position of Director of Sports Nutrition at the University of Florida and was a sport dietitian for the US Olympic Committee where he was fortunate to travel to the 2008 Olympics as a sport dietitian. Bob is known to think outside the box and politely challenge the "why's" behind the way things work. These two traits have brought Bob's work to the attention of many high caliber athletes and coaches and fellow health professionals. He is considered to be a thought provoking sport dietitian who constantly strives for excellence in his work with athletes by always attempting to leave no stone unturned when it comes to improving performance.

Currently, Bob provides sports nutrition services to all types of athletes including endurance, strength, power and aesthetic/skills based through his company, Fuel4mance (www.fuel4mance.com). In addition to his sport nutrition emphasis, Bob is one of the foremost experts on strength training for endurance athletes and holds the NSCA Certified Strength and Conditioning Specialist certification. He is also a USA Triathlon Level III Elite Coach, having worked with Susan Williams, 2004 Olympic Triathlon Bronze Medalist, as her strength coach and sport dietitian, as coach and sport dietitian to Sarah Haskins, 2008 Olympian in triathlon, and coach and sport dietitian of Jasmine Oeinck, 2009 Elite National Champion triathlete. In 2009, Bob teamed up with Susan Williams to provide professional, age-group and junior triathlon coaching through their company, Elite Multisport Coaching (www. teamemc.com).

Practicing what he preaches, Bob is a competitive athlete himself. Growing up playing soccer for 18 years, he shifted his focus to endurance competitions in 1993 off of a dare and has not looked back since. He has competed in hundreds of multi-sport races, most notably six Ironman races, the Boston Marathon, the Leadville 100 mile mountain bike race and the Leadville 100 mile trail run. In 2009 he became a Leadman, completing a series of ultra-endurance events that included a marathon, 50 mile mountain bike race, 50 mile trail run, 100 mile mountain bike race, 10 kilometer run and 100 mile run, all in a span of 7 weeks at altitudes of 10,200 feet and above. The longer and more challenging the endeavor, the better as Bob truly believes in taking his body to the physical, mental and nutritional boundaries. He is truly a "walk the talk" sport dietitian and has a keen understanding for the physical, mental and nutritional components that it takes to be a successful athlete.

Appendix
Metabolic Testing Centers in the United States

USING THIS DOCUMENT

Specific questions were asked to individuals who provide metabolic testing and the answers that you will see throughout this document are based on the following questions:

1. What type of metabolic testing do you offer?

2. What type of metabolic cart do you use and does it analyze oxygen and carbon dioxide.

3. Does your metabolic cart provide a data sheet that can be interpreted and manipulated in addition to the machine's interpretation?

4. Who is the person administering the testing and what are their qualifications?

5. What protocols are used for the metabolic testing?

6. What is the location of the testing?

7. What is the price of the testing and is there a discount provided to USA Triathlon members and coaches?

8. Is there any additional information you would like to share?

Please note each question with the accompanying number assigned to it as you peruse this document.

DISCLAIMER

The information in this document has been collected by Bob Seebohar of Fuel-4mance, LLC and does not represent any endorsement to any facility or person. The information was collected to provide a service to the sport community and has been obtained in an effort to provide athletes and coaches locations where metabolic testing is performed. There are a total of 27 facilities.

Coaches and athletes should contact the person and/or facility for more information. Bob Seebohar is not responsible for misinformation or anything beyond the distribution of this document.

METABOLIC TESTING LOCATIONS CAN BE FOUND ALPHABETICALLY BY STATE

California (3)

1. VO2, RMR

2. New Leaf (MedGraphics VO2000), yes

3. Yes

4. n/a

5. Ability to run any desired protocols on Treadmill, CompuTrainer

6. Location of testing. TRIFIT Club & Studios & TRIFIT MultiSport 2425 Colorado Ave #120 Santa Monica, CA 90404. www.TriFitLA.com; www.TriFitMultisport.com

7. Contact for cost information

8. TRIFIT Club & Studios is the only full service 20,000 square foot health club in Santa Monica that was created by and for MultiSport athletes.

---

1. Cycling VO2, BMR Testing

2. Parvo Medics, yes.

3. We have qualified physiologists that analyze the data and go over results following the assessment. We will provide a complete consultation to help you understand the results and how to apply them to your fitness or training program.

4. Lab technicians/sports physiologists with a exercise physiology degree administer the tests. The consultation is performed by a qualified sports physiologist, with a MSc in Physiology, or an equivalent qualification.

5. Protocols are individualized based on each client.

   • Cycling economy at sub-maximal power

- Two thresholds used to design training intensities and zones for power and/or heart rate.

- Peak Power • Power to Weight Ratio • Absolute and Relative VO2max • Running economy at sub-maximal power

- Two thresholds used to design training intensities and zones for pace and/or heart rate.

- Peak Velocity

- Absolute and Relative VO2max

6. Location of testing- Endurance Performance Training Center (www.enduranceptc.com);

- 747 Front St., SF, CA 94111

- 8 Madrona St., Mill Valley, 94949

7. Cost of testing and any discounts for USAT members/coaches. $249 for fitness assessments $199 for BMR

---

1. Computrainer currently, treadmill coming.

2. New Leaf, yes

3. Yes

4. Registered Dietitian, certified personal trainer

5. Computrainer with heart rate , RPE, and watts

6. www.teamrevolutionscycling.com, Folson, CA

7. Cost of testing and any discounts for USAT members/coaches. $150.00 - not a big fan of the resting test but will offer it

Colorado (3)

1. Indirect calorimetry to determine metabolic efficiency, incremental to determine crossover point and continuous for race specific nutrition planning.

2. Parvomedics True One metabolic cart

3. Yes

4. Bob Seebohar, MS, RD, CSSD, CSCS; BS-Exercise and Sport Science, MS-Health and Exercise Science, MS-Food Science and Human Nutrition; exercise physiologist, USAT Level III Elite Coach, Registered Dietitian and former US Olympic Committee Sport Dietitian

5. Customized to the specific test.

6. Fuel4mance, LLC. Littleton/Denver, Colorado. coachbob@fuel4mance.com;

303-242-7955.

7. Contact for information.

8. All results are interpreted by a nationally known sport dietitian, elite triathlon coach and exercise physiologist. Interpretations are comprehensive and include exercise and nutrition prescriptions.

---

1. Full range

2. Parvo Medics, yes

3. Yes

4. Alan Couzens, exercise physiologist

5. Contact for more information

6. Endurance Corner, Boulder, Colorado

7. alan@endurancecorner.com; gordon@endurancecorner.com

---

1. Indirect calorimetry (FUEL test), VO2 max

2. Sensormedics Encore and Sensormedics Vmax 229, both O2 and CO2 measured in both systems.

3. Yes and is for every test, and proper calibration is performed for every test.

4. Paul Kammermeier, MS (exercise physiologist), Adam St. Pierre, MS (exercise physiologist), Neal Henderson, MS (exercise physiologist)

5. Four minute stages for FUEL test, indirect calorimetry (FUEL) data uses only last 2 minutes of each stage.

6. Boulder Center for Sports Medicine in Boulder, CO and occasionally off-site. www.bch.org/sportsmedicine or (303) 441-2285

7. $150, $200, $250 depending on lactate, LT/VO2, or FUEL (LT, indirect calorimetry, and VO2max)

8. BCSM is a CLIA certified laboratory and also performs diagnostic testing and EKG evaluations when appropriate. All results consultations include consultation with an exercise physiologist with coaching experience and all FUEL tests also have consultation with registered dietitian with sports nutrition experience.

Florida (2)

1. RMR, Energy Assessment

2. Parvo Medics TrueOne 2400 (analyzes O2 and CO2) and Korr CardioCoach Plus

3. Yes, Only the TruMax

4. Jeff Plasschaert - Exercise Physiologist MS, CSCS, USAT, USAC

5. n/a

6. UF & Shands Sports Performance Center (www.ufsportsperformance.com) Gainesville, Florida

7. Metabolic Rate Test $50, $40 for follow-up tests. Energy Assessment Test $100

---

1. VO2 max and Resting Metabolic Rate

2. Sensor Medics

3. Yes

4. We have a small group of Exercise physiologists holding a Master's Degree along with a reputable certification. Our main Human Performance Lab Exercise Physiologist's name is Sharlyne Rivera, MA, ACSM HFI, RRCA.

5. Protocols used. We can and do use several depending on the population sample. However, with triathletes we use USOC protocol.

6. Location of testing. USA National Training Center Human Performance Lab, Clermont, Florida. Carol Kneller, 352-241-7144 x4202, carol.kneller@orlandohealth.com

7. Cost of testing and any discounts for USAT members/coaches. VO2 max = 150.00, RMR and body composition=100.00; any testing done in a package of 3 or more is discounted 15%.

Idaho (1)

1. RMR, V02 Submax, V02 Max

2. KORR MetaCheck, KORR Cardio Coach

3. Yes, with additional monitor software

4. Chris Baker, B.S. Sports Science, B.S. Nutrition, M.S. Exercise Physiology, USAS/USAC/USAT cerified coach, NASM Personal Trainer

5. ACSM protocol. Depends on test. (use both a computrainer and treadmill)

6. Coeur D'Alene, ID

7. $125 V02, $75 RMR, both for $150

8. www.train4endurance.com

Illinois (1)

1. New Leaf

2. Yes

3. On request raw values can be provided, in my past life I specialized in reporting and data manipulation, so if there is specific analysis that is requested this can be done without too much hassle (technology used, Excel, Crystal Reports, Oracle etc.)

4. Annette Jonker, USAT Coach Level 1

5. Walk, run, bike (stationary and CompuTrainer for power based numbers), protocol specific to client.

6. My Fitness Company, LLC 2103 N Western Ave, Chicago, IL 60647 773-252-0252

7. Cost-please enquire, 20% discount for USAT members (not to be combined with any other discounts or special rates), additional discount for coaches.

Massachusetts (2)

1. VO2max, steady state VO2 and substrate metabolism, resting metabolism

2. Parvomedics True One metabolic cart

3. Yes

4. Jeff Godin, Ph.D. 15 years experience administering metabolic tests

5. Depends on what the objective is, generally 4 minutes stages for lactate threshold testing, one minute stages for VO2max, during steady state metabolism test subject exercises for 15 minutes at predetermined workload without VO2 measurement, then an addition 15 minutes with VO2 measurement. Depending on the athlete and the goals of the testing we may test after a long ride or run to see the effects of prolonged exercise rather than what is happening during the early stages of exercise.

6. Blackstone Valley Human Performance, 210 Worcester Street, North Grafton, MA 01536

7. VO2max test $110.00, steady state exercise test $150.00

---

1. Resting metabolic rate, VO2 max

2. New leaf, yes

3. Yes

4. Ali Winslow, MS, USAT Level II coach, NASM CPT/IFS, Pilates certified; Vic Brown, MS, USAT Level I coach, CSCS, ATC

5. Depends on the mode, treadmill or bike.

6. www.bostonperformancecoaching.com

7. Full metabolic profile, $340.

8. We offer a 30 minute meeting with one of our coaches after the test. We also offer a meeting with our nutritionist as well as our physical therapists.

Missouri (1)

1. Resting (provides nutrition info) and Exercise (provides intensity info)

2. New Leaf, analyzes both O2 uptake and CO2 production

3. Yes, the raw data can be manipulated to the discretion of the administrator, if necessary

4. Testing is administered by the fitness staff at MCC Maple Woods Fitness Center.

   • Each instructor has a minimum of a B.S. in Exercise Science or related field.

5. Protocols begin at an unfit/sedentary walker. They increase to an elite runner. Protocols may be modified to the tester's discretion during the assessment, if necessary.

6. MCC Maple Woods Fitness Center, 3100 NE 83rd St, Ste 2600, KC, MO 64119 http:// mcckc.edu/maplewoods/fitness/

7. Mandatory kit purchase at first test, required $50; all tests are $25 per test 8. Any other information that is pertinent to this. Testing can be done during any of our operating hours, seven days a week. There are some conditions to be met prior to testing time.

Montana (1)

1. Basal, VE, VO2, VCO2, Fat/Carb ratios, caloric burn, aerobic base (highest HR at 50% fat, 50% carb utilization)

2. New Leaf system, analyzes oxygen and carbon dioxide.

3. Only manipulated in "cow files".

4. Gene Lemelin

5. Stage protocols

6. Peak Health and Wellness Center 1800 Benefis Ct. Great Fall, Montana 59405, 406-727-7325

7. Cost of testing and any discounts for USAT members/coaches.

   • Initial RMR. $85, follow up assessments are $75

   • Initial EMR $125, follow up assessments are $85

I take 10% off initial assessments as a corporate rate (3 or more clients purchasing assessments)

New York (3)

1. Vo2 max, ventilatory threshold testing, substrate utilization testing (metabolic efficiency)

2. New Leaf; it does analyze and report O2 and CO2 use

3. Yes, the cart does provide this information; you can export a raw data sheet and re-interpret, or graph it in any way you want

4. Darian Silk, MSc in Exercise Physiology and Certified Exercise Physiologist

5. Various, depending on client needs and ability levels, can be done on a treadmill, cybex bike, computrainer with client's own bike

6. Altheus Health and Sport, 2 Clinton Ave., Rye, NY, 10580; ph: 914-921-3044; fx: 914-921-0829; email: info@altheus.net; web: www.altheus.net

7. One of : VO2, VT or metabolic efficiency test : $150 Various discounts available with training or coaching package purchase.

---

1. Gas exchange

2. New Leaf PAS measure both O2 & CO2.

3. n/a

4. David Schneider, USAT Level 2 Coach

5. Treadmill & Bike (on Computrainer)

6. Floral Park, NY. On the border of Queens & Nassau, about 30 minutes outside of Manhatten

7. Bike test - $150. Run test - $125. 20% discount for USAT members

---

1. VO2 Max, resting metabolic, and substrate utilization.

2. Medgraphics CPX D for base location and Medgraphics VO2000 for travel.

3. Both systems measure CO2. I provide customized reports and interpret the data as I see fit.

4. Doug Bush, Bachelors of Science in Exercise Physiology with a concentration in Sports Nutrition. Level II USAT and Level I (Elite) USAT coaching certifications.

5. Bruce, Balke, and many customized

6. Ellicottville, NY. Buffalo, NY. Rochester, NY. Syracuse, NY. Elmira, NY. New Paltz, NY. Tenafly, NJ. Pittsburgh, PA.

7. Threshold/VO2 - $120 single sport, $195. Substrate Utilization - $120 Resting Metabolic - $100

8. Referral fees and discounts are provide to coaches for their athletes.

North Carolina (2)

1. 12 lead EKG, gas exchange.

2. Parvomedics. Analyzes both O2 and CO2.

3. Our physiologists are creating interpretation reports from the Parvo data and counseling athletes through those written results immediately after the test completion.

EKG data will be read and given to the athlete as well.

4. The staff includes a cardiac rehab nurse or cardiologist (depending on risk stratification of the subject) and one or two exercise physiologists. At least one of the physiologists is a USA Triathlon coach.

5. Our protocols will be individualized for the athletes, generally a 5 minute warm up at a jog and maxing out at 6, 7, 8 or 9 miles per hour (depending on the athletes' race pace). Once the max speed is reached, we begin increasing the incline 0.5% every 30 seconds until athlete max is reached.

6. The UNC Performance Lab is located within the UNC Wellness Center. Betty Matteson (919-843-2154, ematteson@unch.unc.edu).

7. We are charging $200 for a nurse administered test and $250 for physician administered.

8. We can offer a 15% discount to USAT coaches and members, with proof of membership.

---

1. Maximal oxygen consumption, metabolic thresholds (with lactate threshold), resting metabolic rate, calorie/substrate utilization during exercise.

2. Vacumed mini CPX analyzes O2 and CO2

3. Our lab interprets all raw data and creates a custom results page for each client. All results are based upon raw data all calculations are cross checked with multiple measures of metabolism.

4. Chris Eschbach, Ph.D., ACSM-HFS; Dr. Eschbach, Associate Professor of Exercise and Sport Science at Meredith College; Chris Newport, ACSM-HFS, USAT level 2

   • A competitive endurance athlete with education in exercise science, nutrition, and business.

5. Specific to individual client. 6. Meredith College, Raleigh, NC 7. http://www.meredith.edu/hess/lab/testing_specifics.htm 8. Website: www.humanperformancetesting.com

Oregon (1)

1. Resting metabolic rate, exercise testing

2. New Leaf Metabolic Cart, analyzes oxygen and carbon dioxide.

3. I will exclusively use the raw data to establish optimal training intensities and nutritional planning for training sessions as well as race day nutritional plans.

4. Mark Kendall, USA Triathlon Level II, USA Cycling Level 2, Masters Swimming Coach, NSCA: CSCS

5. Typically an incremental method (wattage for bike, pace and incline for running) with steady state testing and numbers established prior to last big key workout (for

practice purposes) 3-4 weeks out from event.

6. 1722 NW Portland, Studio #112, Portland, OR 97239, 503-332-8710, mark@speedshotracing.com, www.speedshotracing.com

7. $200 for combination RMR, exercise or bike and run testing. No discounts set-up but happy to establish a referral discount for other coaches.

South Carolina (1)

1. RMR (Resting Metabolic Rate), VO2 max/sub max test and what we call a Metabolic Profile Assessment (the combination of both)

2. Cardio Coach PLUS from KORR. It does analyze both O2 and CO2.

3. Yes.

4. Masters in Exercise and Sport Science.

5. Steady state test or a modified Balke protocol 95% of the time.

6. TEMPO Indoor Cycling, 1123 Queensborough Blvd, Suite 100, Mt. Pleasant, SC 29464, 843-884-4822, www.tempoindoorcycling.com

7. RMR, $109; USAT members/coaches, $99: VO2max/submax, $145: USAT members/ coaches, $129: Metabolic profile assessment, $239; USAT members/coaches, $199.

Texas (1)

1. New leaf and cardio coach

2. Oxygen and carbon dioxide

3. Yes

4. Ahmed Zaher.

5. We ask the athlete to get ready for the test as if he/she are doing a speed workout, this way they don't hurt themselves during the test but also so that they don't change their diet, this way we can get the most accurate data possible.

6. Dallas, Texas. Ahmed Zaher, 214-738-8737, www.playtri.com 7. $150 including analysis and tools to help improve your personal metabolic system.

Washington (2)

1. VO2 max, Resting Metabolic Rate

2. New Leaf Metabolic Cart - O2 and CO2

3. Yes.

4. David Fleischhauer. BS in Exercise Science, FaCT certified.

5. FaCT Protocol for Lactate Testing. VO2 max: Standard ramp test with 2 minute steps

on either computrainer or treadmill.

6. Herriott Sports Performance - 101 Nickerson St #150 Seattle, WA 98109

7. $125 for VO2 max

---

1. VO2 Active Metabolic Fitness Testing & Resting Metabolic Rate

2. New Leaf Cart measures both O2 & CO2

3. Yes–if need be.

4. Annelise DiGiacomo with INFITNESS is a Certified Metabolic Specialist, ACSM Certified Health Fitness Specialist, USA Cycling & USAT Triathlon Certified Coach and a Heart Zones Master Trainer.

5. Tests are performed on a treadmill or bicycle and depending on current fitness level, walking with incline or running protocols will be used if treadmill test and if on a bike, different % of watts increase will be used. Power/Watts are measured during cycling tests. The Metabolic VO2 Fitness Assessment takes approximately 10 – 15 minutes, however, I ask to expect about 45 – 60 minutes total assessment time with set-up, evaluation, and explanation of test results. During the test, exercise intensity measured in either watts or speed is increased every minute while data is provided every 15 seconds. Tests can be done on other cardio equipment as well, ie; rower, elliptical, arm ergometer, Wave, plus more.

6. The machine & equipment I have is a portable system and so I am able to provide testing to various locations within the greater Puget Sound area of Seattle and Eastside Communities. Ongoing testing is provided in a small studio setting in Issaquah and Bellevue

7. All testing pricing & packages may be found on my website. I will provide up to a 25% discount to USAT members and coaches.

8. Through Heart Zones USA, (www.heartzones.com) we have several testing centers across the US providing the same type of testing, zone training and periodized programs for fitness, health and performance. Other locations include: Sacramento California, Chicago, and Pennsylvania. Our locations are continuing to grow and expand into other areas as well.

Wisconsin (3)

1. Resting, anaerobic threshold, VO2 max

2. Cortex MetaLyzer 3B, analyzes O2 and CO2

3. Yes.

4. Bob Hanisch, Master's degree Exercise Physiology from Columbia University in NY city. Certified coach USAT and USAC. Adjunct Graduate faculty in the Dietetic Department for Mount Mary College teaching Exercise Physiology as well as Nutrition in Sports and Fitness.

5. Typical treadmill and CompuTrainer protocols with 3 or 4 minute stages depending on including lactate. Individualize to each person ability and for cycling their body weight.

6. 4125 N. 124th Street, Suite A Brookfield WI 53005, phone: 262.439.8601, email: bob@peakperformancepros.com

7. RMR: $125, Threshold: $165, Max: $175, Discounts members 10%, coaches 20%. 8. Results are always discussed so the individual understands what they mean and how to use it. Free follow up questions are encouraged after the evaluation is completed and discussed.

---

1. VO2max AND RMR

2. O2, CARDIOCOACH PLUS

3. Yes.

4. BS-Kinesiology, MA-Exercise Physiology, NSCA-CSCS, USAT Level I

5. Customized.

6. Verona, WI

7. $130 FOR TEST, 10% FOR USAT

8. www.sbrcoaching.com, 608-695-8942

---

1. VO2 Peak, SubMax, RMR.

2. NewLeaf P.A.S.

3. Yes.

4. Angie Sturtevant - Over 15 years experience in coaching, training and assess- ment. USAC Elite Level 1 Cycling Coach; USAC Power Based Cycling Coach; USAT Triathlon Coach; Saris Cycling Group-CycleOps Power Education Director & Master Training Specialist; Evolve Metabolic Testing Specialist; ACE/AFAA Personal Trainer & Con- tinuing Education Provider

5. Various protocols based on test, testee, health history and goals. 6. Madison, WI, www.vo2test.com 7. RMR - $85; VO2 $140-$175, depending upon goal/test proto- col required